MEDICINE IN OLD AGE

MEDICINE IN OLD AGE

Second edition

Articles from the *British Medical Journal*

Published by the British Medical Association
Tavistock Square, London WC1H 9JR

First published 1978
Second Edition 1985

British Library Cataloguing in Publication Data

Medicine in old age.—2nd ed.
  1. Geriatrics
  I. British Medical Association
  618.97   RC952

ISBN 0-7279-0112-5

Printed in Great Britain by the
University Press, Cambridge

Contents

Note
Due to an error the page
numbers on pages 46, 47
and 91 have not been
printed.

Dementia in the elderly: diagnosis and assessment

TOM ARIE

Few patients are so taxing to doctors as the confused and demented. No other condition generates so much crisis, irritability, and interprofessional friction. Dementia is common: about 10% of old people are demented, half of them severely, and in the over 80s this proportion rises to more than one in five. Most are women because, among the very old, they outnumber men by over two to one. There will be even more old people with dementia as the number of the very old continues to increase rapidly. Until recently, with some outstanding exceptions, few doctors took any interest in dementia. Yet an average general practitioner is likely to have 30-40 demented patients on his list, and every general practitioner knows that the demands made by many of these patients are out of proportion to their numbers, not least because their problems often present as crises.

The reasons why the "psychogeriatric crisis" is so common are not difficult to see, and one reason is that, of the important conditions among elderly patients living at home, dementia is the one that their general practitioners are least likely to be aware of. In a study conducted in Edinburgh Williamson *et al* found that over 80% of moderately or severely demented old people were not known to be so by their general practitioners. As these patients rarely seek medical help for themselves it is not surprising that crises occur when their disabilities impinge on others or are "unmasked" by the death of a spouse or the marriage of a daughter. Preventive measures must be based on the general practice team, although the high rate of admission of old people to hospital provides a valuable opportunity to screen the mental function of the patient.

Causes of dementia

Dementia in the elderly is an acquired global disruption of higher mental function. It affects in varying degree personality, memory, behaviour, emotion, skill, intelligence, and, often, speech and causes impairment of the ability to learn new responses and thus to adapt to a changing environment. Most dementias are progressive. In dementia consciousness is unimpaired, but superimposed confusional states are common, and if they occur their cause must be sought. Often an astonishing degree of function may be preserved provided that the old person remains in a constant environment with which she is familiar and new demands on her are not great. Even so, such preservation is always precarious, depending on a constancy and security that are unlikely to last long.

Alzheimer's and multi-infarct dementia

Dementia is of two main types, Alzheimer (senile) and multi-infarct. Alzheimer's dementia is characterised by degeneration of the parenchymatous tissue of the brain, the rate and extent of which is determined partly but not wholly genetically. Alzheimer dementias that develop late – that is, in the late 70s – generally have a more benign course with longer survival and less serious structural and biochemical deficits than those of younger patients, and genetic factors also seem less important. In multi-infarct dementia the brain substance degenerates as the result of impaired blood supply and infarction causes disseminated softenings. In Alzheimer's dementia the surface of the brain shrinks, the sulci are widened, and the ventricles are dilated: usually, the temporal lobes are particularly affected. Other rare types of presenile dementia include: Pick's disease, affecting chiefly the frontal lobes; Jakob-Creutzfeldt disease, which usually runs a rapid course and, though rare, is of great theoretical importance through having been shown to be due to a transmissible agent; and Huntington's chorea, with an autosomal dominant inheritance, the gross clinical manifestations of which are only rarely delayed until late life.

By contrast, in multi-infarct dementia the nature of the deficit depends on the site of damage: thus a patient may have brain damage without dementia but dementia is likely when a substantial volume of brain has been destroyed. Whereas senile dementia generally follows a steady downhill course, a "step by step" course is typical in multi-infarct dementia, often with relatively lucid intervals. During these intervals the patient may have so much insight into his own predicament that his plight is one of the most

2

pitiful in medicine. The patient often has a shallow lability of mood in which he is laughing at one moment and crying the next. This makes it easy to miss the depressive state that is common in these patients and which may respond to antidepressant drugs or electroplexy. A history of hypertension and strokes is common. Epilepsy is much more common in multi-infarct dementia than in senile dementia.

Some patients have senile and multi-infarct brain damage simultaneously as both are common. Wandering, incontinence, and impaired capacity for self care are features of both conditions, as are paranoid developments; visual hallucinations are more characteristic of multi-infarct dementia. Neuropathological studies have confirmed that clinical distinction between the two types of dementia is fairly accurate and that a relation exists between the characteristic histological changes in the brain in senile dementia, including "senile plaques," "neurofibrillary tangles," and deficits in several neurotransmitters (especially cholinergic) and its clinical severity. Though the expectation of life for both groups is less than normal for their age, it appears to be increasing – with obvious consequences for the use of beds and other resources.

Other causes of dementia

Other conditions may lead to dementia, but, in the absence of specific evidence, most are not common causes. These are: tumours; subdural haematomas; giant aneurysms; trauma, including the chronic trauma of boxers; syphilis and non-syphilitic inflammatory disease; chronic alcoholism; normal pressure or communicating hydrocephalus; myxoedema; vitamin B_{12} deficiency; chronic epilepsy; carcinomatosis; and systemic lupus.

Amnestic states

Amnestic states, the most common of which is Korsakoff's psychosis of chronic alcoholics, are characterised by a specific defect in the recent memory without the damage to personality, intelligence, and emotion that is suffered in dementia. The degree to which the intelligence is spared is shown by the ingenuity of the confabulation that fills the deficit of memory. The syndrome may present acutely or subacutely as a confusional state with the ataxia, eye signs (most commonly nystagmus), and peripheral neuritis of Wernicke's encephalopathy. The neurological features of thiamine deficiency almost always respond quite rapidly to parenteral vitamins in high dosage, but the mental changes improve more slowly and not always completely.

3

Acute confusional states

Almost any physical, social, or psychological disturbance in an old person may produce a confusional state. In multi-infarct dementia such acute episodes are especially common, but in general the more severe the underlying dementia the more readily may an acute confusional episode be precipitated. Moreover, the more demented the patient the less specific may be the precipitants of the confusional state.

Why does dementia so often present as a crisis?

Obviously, if a doctor does not know that an elderly patient is demented, that patient is more likely suddenly to catch him unawares than one for whom measures of support have already been undertaken. Crises are inconvenient, unpleasant, and difficult to deal with calmly (for anxiety is easily communicated) but are inherent in this work, and, although they cannot be wholly "organised away," insight into their genesis should help to make them more intelligible, less common, and perhaps even more bearable. The following rough classification is suggested.

Firstly, something has happened to the patient, which may be a further stage in the process of dementing – for instance, a stroke (in the case of multi-infarct dementia) or an intercurrent illness. Often such a change will present as acute confusion.

Secondly, something has happened in the environment, such as a sudden change in the people relied on for support – for instance, the main caring relative has been admitted to hospital or has died or a patient who lives alone has suddenly been discharged from hospital without any forethought about her capacity to cope. Often the event is less straightforward: tolerance of the old person may snap because of a marital row in the family caring for her, or the family may become anxious about the effect a confused old lady is having on a teenager who is working for exams.

Thirdly, "enough is enough": people can take so much and then no more, particularly when no end is in sight. Thus the old lady may wander out of her house in her underclothes and be cheerfully fielded back, but when she has done so a second, a third, or a 10th time tolerance may break, especially if the caring services have not responded adequately.

Fourthly, the crisis may be a manipulation of the caring system. This may arise for one or more of the following reasons.

Local services may be poor. If it is impossible, or thought to be impossible, to get help from local services by making requests calmly and reasonably, families and general practitioners will understandably resort to declaring an emergency. It follows that when a service has begun to function well the rate of crisis referrals invariably falls (and referrals as a whole increase).

Ignorance may result in many doctors and social workers being unable to formulate a "psychogeriatric" problem in any terms other than the need to get it instantly off their hands. They are most unlikely to have had any training in these matters—a state of affairs that is at last improving. A subcategory of this group is those who become irritable and resentful when asked to deal with anything but a straightforward somatic problem.

Guilt may give rise to the "Monday morning syndrome," a common manifestation that is familiar to many general practitioners, psychiatrists, geriatricians, and their secretaries. An old lady, often coping quite well, but not perfectly, is living alone, and her children come for their quarterly Sunday visit. They see she could do with some extra care but are unable or unwilling to provide it themselves. They telephone the general practitioner "first thing on Monday morning" to say that "something must be done."

The preventive crisis or the "Friday afternoon crisis," paradoxically an example of forethought (though this is rarely carried over into the general management), derives from the fact that the relatives or professional attendants who are concerned with the patient are planning to go away for the weekend.

This list oversimplifies: the genesis of crisis is always multifactorial.

Assessment

An organic psychiatric syndrome should always be assessed initially at home because it is an old person's capacity to function in her normal surroundings that needs to be assessed. In addition, assessment at home makes it possible to see the physical surroundings and often to suggest practical changes in the domestic arrangements. Members of the family and neighbours should be interviewed, and I cannot overemphasise that reliable histories obtained from others are paramount in assessing dementia. It often helps if a social worker is present so that discussion and joint decisions can take place on the spot. On the other hand, it may be more appropriate for the health visitor or district nurse to accompany the general practitioner.

It is always wise to inquire whether the patient is already known to the social services department as general practitioners are not always notified when confused old people are referred directly to the social services by relatives or neighbours. If the initial assessment indicates that specialist help may be needed it is usually preferable for the specialist also to see the patient at home.

The assessment begins with a history from a relative, neighbour, or other informant. I prefer to obtain this before I meet the patient, who is often in another room and unaware of one's arrival. Once one has engaged the attention of a demented person it is often difficult to disengage again – for example, if you leave to talk to a relative the patient is likely to become anxious, wondering what you are up to, and to interrupt with perseverant, repetitive questioning and by repeatedly coming back into the room. The history from the relative usually helps direct subsequent interviews with the patient towards the roots of the problem.

The assessment itself follows the general principles of physical and mental examination. The following points should be noted routinely.

General appearance

Is the patient's general appearance compatible with the history?
Do the mental and physical states more or less match each other?
Are any of the following present: anaemia, myxoedema, or neurological and locomotor deficits?
Is the patient deaf (and if so, using a deaf aid?) or blind?
Is there chestiness or heart failure?
Is she smelly or wet?

State of the household

If the old person lives alone the state of her home will often be the best measure of her capacity for self care (but one must establish what help she receives from others.) The kitchen and contents of the larder are particularly eloquent. What was the last meal? How much of it has been eaten? Is there an accumulation of bottles? More generally, is the place clean and warm? Has hygiene has been grossly neglected? Has the bed been slept in?

Mental examination

The mental examination follows standard lines but is particularly aimed at assessing cognitive functions, largely by ascertaining the patient's grasp of the material of everyday life. The examination must be unhurried, and the patient will need a few moments to take in what is happening. A strange man suddenly appearing off the street and immediately asking, "What is the name of the prime minister?" is likely either to put the final touch to the patient's confusion or to convince her that she has fallen into the hands of a madman. One should explain carefully who one is. I usually ask the patient to remember my name, which I then repeat to her, explaining that I will ask her to repeat it later "because I want to see how good your memory is." The questioning should develop naturally from the opening remarks and, so far as possible, resemble a normal conversation. The interview will cover personal details such as the patient's age, date of birth, address, etc, and general matters. A short series of questions can detect and roughly measure intellectual impairment. A typical series would contain 10 questions, such as, in brief: Town? Address? Date? Month? Year? Age? Year of birth? Month of birth? Prime minister? Previous prime minister? You should always ask the questions, never simply assume the answers, and record the results for comparison with future (or previous) testing. Finally, simple tests of cortical function – that is, dysphasia and dyspraxia – should be done.

Basis of management

At the end of the assessment, as well as having a good idea of the mental state, the doctor should be able to answer the following questions, on which the subsequent management largely depends:

Does the patient live alone?

How long has it been since she was "normal" and competent? *How* did the change in her begin and was it sudden or gradual? Did it coincide with any event – for example, injury, illness, or bereavement?

What course has the disability taken since then? Has it been steady or intermittent?

Is the patient mobile? Does she go out of the house?

What can she do for herself? Can she use the toilet, wash, dress, clean, shop, or cook?

What odd or undesirable behaviour does she have? Does she wander? Is she incontinent? Is she up at night? Does she make paranoid accusations? Is she agressive or destructive?

What resources – for example, relatives, friends, money – are available?

What services are already concerned?

Which consultant to call?

If a specialist is needed to give further help with either the home assessment or possible hospital admission a psychiatrist should be called if the problem is primarily disturbed behaviour. If the problem is primarily physical illness or decrepitude the geriatrician should be called. A full description of these services can be found in two chapters of *Psychiatry of Late Life*,[1,2] which also contains a reprint of a series of guidelines on division of responsibility officially agreed by geriatricians and psychiatrists. One test of the quality of a district service for old people is whether it makes much difference if the "wrong" specialist is called: in a good service the geriatrician and psychiatrist will be accustomed to working together and taking patients from each other.

If, even with the help of a specialist, the home assessment does not enable you to decide whether the disability is primarily medical or psychiatric, or if further assessment or care will need both general medical and psychiatric skills, the patient may be admitted to a psychogeriatric assessment unit or joint patient unit or, best of all, to a department jointly staffed by geriatric physicians and psychiatrists, such as we have in Nottingham.

Investigations

In most cases a diagnosis of dementia, senile or multi-infarct, can be made at the patient's home. In a very elderly person a history of progressive deterioration over months or years is so typical that when it coincides with the clinical findings, both physical and mental, the diagnosis can be regarded as conclusive. In such patients it is not necessary to pursue elaborate investigations designed to find one of the rare and so called reversible causes of dementia when clinical evidence of them – for example, anaemia, hypothyroidism, papilloedema, or other abnormal neurological signs – is not present. The most fashionable "reversible" causes of dementia are: hypothyroidism, vitamin B_{12} deficiency, and normal pressure hydrocephalus, which should be considered especially in patients with a history of subarachnoid haemorrhage or meningitis. But in patients with established dementia and a long history of progressive deterioration treatment of the first two of these conditions is most unlikely to improve the mental state of the patient in any way. The same pessimistic view may ultimately be shown to apply to treatment for normal pressure hydrocephalus with its triad of dementia, gait disturbance, and incontinence, which has the added hazard of the remedial operation. In most patients, who will be in their 80s, home assessment will suffice to reach a conclusion, and the issue will then turn on management rather than on further investigation. (Research is another matter, and with the availability of non-invasive techniques routine full investigation of even very aged dements in a few centres should be feasible and worth while.)

Further observations or fuller investigations

In the following groups a diagnosis of dementia based on the history and initial examination alone should not be regarded as conclusive: (*a*) patients who have a history or any features suggestive of depressive illness; (*b*) all patients under 70 unless there is an obvious – for example, cerebrovascular – cause; (*c*) patients of any age whose history is atypical or uncertain – for example, a course that has been too short, unusually rapid, or atypically intermittent; (*d*) patients in whom there are other unusual features – for example, recent injury, intercurrent illness, alcoholism, or drug abuse – and patients with unexplained physical findings or whose mental state on examination is greatly at variance with the history; and (*e*) patients in whom one has the feel that they are somehow "not right." The last is hardly a helpful category to others, but psychiatrists working in the field of psychogeriatrics will know what I mean. These patients may turn out to be depressed. Some may ascribe this category, perhaps rightly, to imprecision of thinking or observation.

Further investigation is likely to comprise: measurement of blood count and sedimentation rate; testing for syphilis; estimation of blood sugar, calcium, urea, and electrolyte concentrations; urine analysis; chest and skull radiography; tests of thyroid function; estimation of serum vitamin B_{12} and folate; and tests of liver function, especially if there is evidence of alcoholism. Nowadays, the test for syphilis is not really expected to yield a result of relevance to the patient: the occasional positive result is almost always incidental to, rather than the cause of, the dementia and is one of the "persistent positives" that occur among thoroughly treated cases of syphilis. We perform the above tests routinely on most inpatients, although not all of our inpatients are demented and many have other mental disorders and acute confusional states. Other laboratory tests may be made necessary by specific findings.

Psychological tests may sometimes help with specific deficits, though in our experience they are more helpful in providing a baseline against which to measure change. Electroencephalography is likely merely to confirm the presence of diffuse abnormality in severely demented patients, while appearing normal in the mild or uncertain case. Examination of the cerebrospinal fluid is scarcely ever necessary in demented elderly patients: the main indications are suspected syphilis or some other infective process.

When to perform computed tomography?

The availability of non-invasive computed tomography is a major innovation. Isotope scanning is often more accessible but less discriminating. Newer techniques of imaging, such as nuclear magnetic resonance and positron emission tomography, are full of promise but not yet generally available. Computed tomography is valuable in displaying space occupying lesions, haemorrhages, infarcts, and cortical atrophy. Computed tomography is neither feasible nor necessary (except for research) in the investigation of every elderly patient in whom the history and clinical picture are typical of dementia.

Two categories of apparently demented patients should normally have computed tomography. Firstly, the "young" – that is, under 70 or 75 – and those who have no obvious vascular or other cause for their dementia. This is to confirm the presence of cortical atrophy and exclude other possible lesions, bearing in mind that appearances of atrophy are quite common in aged people who are not demented. Secondly, those with features suggesting that the diagnosis may not be conclusive to give more confidence by finding obvious cortical atrophy or to detect other possible lesions.

The comments in this chapter refer to patients with a typical history and clinical picture of dementia and no specific or unusual features and not to acutely confused patients who may require exhaustive investigation, which will often show remediable lesions. All those patients in whom we have found tumours, subdural haematomas, cysts, etc, have had clinical features that led us to investigate more fully. I cannot recall any patient who, having undergone computed tomography simply as a matter of routine, then surprised us by showing some unsuspected remediable condition: a fortiori it is fair to assume that the results of performing these procedures on very aged typically demented patients would be no different.

[1] Arie T, Jolley D. In: Levy R, Post F, eds. *Psychiatry of late life*. Oxford: Blackwells Scientific Publications, 1982: 222–51.
[2] Hemsi L. In: Levy R, Post F, eds. *Psychiatry of late life*. Oxford: Blackwells Scientific Publications, 1982: 252–87.

Erratum

On page 10 the first group in whom computed tomography is indicated (2nd sentence of 2nd paragraph) should read: "The 'young' — that is, under 70 or 75 — who have no obvious vascular or other cause for their dementia."

Dementia in the elderly: management

TOM ARIE

Most demented people are at home. Dementia greatly increases the likelihood that an old person will eventually need institutional care but it is not in itself grounds for removal from home. Except when short term admission to hospital for investigation or treatment is necessary, the issue turns on the resources and tolerance available as much as on the nature of the disease itself. Thus in most cases the doctor's job is to ensure that all available medical and social sources of help are deployed and to coordinate and monitor their provision.

Can the patient be managed at home?

The old person who lives alone poses the biggest problem. The available services are rarely able to offer anything approaching continuous 24 hour care. Such old people often have to be admitted to hospital not because they need heavy care but simply because someone has to be there to keep an eye on them most of the time – to reassure or gently restrain them if they start to wander off. If they cannot have this care at home, then it is residential, not hospital care that they need. But old people who are being looked after by relatives or friends may pose equally taxing problems. Sometimes the burden of disability or behaviour disorder is such that the doctor may feel it his duty to try to persuade a devoted family to accept that they cannot reasonably be expected to cope with their parent and to help them with their guilt or grief at accepting to institutional care. The cost of caring for an aged relative in terms of stress, and even of lasting damage to such families, may be clearer to the doctor than to the family, who may find it hard to confess it to themselves or each other.

Usually, the old person can continue to be looked after at home, and relatives and friends will often want to continue to do so. Often it is not the immediate burden that makes families despair but the

11

prospect of carrying on indefinitely without relief, without even the expectation of a holiday, or, for that matter, without some recognition by others of the size of the burden that they are carrying. Often the whole burden of caring for an aged parent is carried by only one among many brothers and sisters, often for reasons that are obscure or derive from longstanding family feuds. In these cases the child who is doing the caring may voice so much resentment towards the brothers and sisters who "don't want to know" that the resentment seems to be harder for them to bear than the burden itself. The family's attitude to an old person often seems to owe more to her past personality and behaviour towards them than to the objective burden of her dementia: in other words, whether they like her.

Many families who do not want to give up the care of the old person need reassurance that their difficulties are appreciated and not taken for granted, and "therapeutic listening" will go a long way. But often families are unaware of the services that exist or how to gain access to them – for example, that the old person can be admitted to hospital or an old people's home for a period of relief and that their holiday arrangements can be safeguarded by booking a temporary admission. In addition, medical measures, which are discussed below, can greatly mitigate problems of behaviour.

If the decision is for hospital admission the family must be clear why the patient is being admitted – that is, whether it is for care and not "treatment" or only for short term investigation. Sometimes the family's hopes prove stronger than even the most careful attempts to explain. In a good unit the patient who has been newly admitted, no matter how demented, will go, firstly, to an assessment ward, and only occasionally will a commitment to permanent hospital care be made at the time of first admission.

Is day care likely to help?

Day care may help families and provide an opportunity to assess or treat the patient further. Some demented old people become upset and confused when moved from place to place, which may limit the feasibility of day care for some patients and also restrict the appropriateness of "rotating" admission, which is such a great source of help to many families looking after physically sick old people.

Transport to and from home often causes difficulties: it may be impossible to pick up a patient, even if she can be got up and ready, before the family leave for work; and at the end of the day relatives still have the old person arriving home around the time that they themselves get back weary from work. The family may be given some respite in the evenings by keeping the day patient until after they have had their tea, while she has hers at the day hospital. This generally depends on the family being able to make their own arrangements for collecting her, as transport is rarely available at this time, and on the day hospital being staffed until the appropriate time. Many of these problems are solved when the day hospital has its own minibus and driver. Another scheme provides a "granny-sitting" service in the evenings at some residential homes: by arrangement with the officer in charge families wishing to go out in the evening may leave an aged relative watching the television with other old people. But, again, confused old people may become still more confused by such temporary changes of surroundings.

Can the patients manage their financial affairs?

An important practical aspect of the care of demented old people, often forgotten, is the legal one. Demented people are unlikely to be able to appreciate the nature of their affairs, still less to look after them, and if there are substantial assets the family should be advised to contact the Court of Protection. In these circumstances a power of attorney is inappropriate because the old person is unlikely to be capable of understanding its meaning. The approach to the Court of Protection may be made through a solicitor or to the personal applications branch.* Occasionally, it may be the doctor's duty to contact the court if he has reason to believe that a demented person is being financially exploited.

Informal or compulsory admission?

Only a minority of patients with organic psychosyndromes are admitted to hospital under compulsion, most of them under the Mental Health Act and a few under section 47 of the National Assistance Act. Hard and fast advice on when the use of these powers is justified is impossible to give, and the decision can be taxing. The effects of the Mental Health Act 1983 on the traditional assumption of consent in the "not unwilling" patient, whose capacity to give informed consent is in question, is a focus of current debate. The new powers of guardianship conferred by this Act may prove useful for demented patients.

Paradoxically perhaps, I have, very rarely, used an order to bring in for a temporary relief admission a demented old person being cared for by her family yet refused to do so for a demented old

* Staffordshire House, Store Street, London WC1E 7BP. Telephone: 01-636 6877.

13

person who lives alone and constitutes some danger to herself. This is the result of applying a general criterion: if the old person is unwilling to enter hospital because of a clear wish to remain at home and, in expressing this, displays at least a reasonable awareness of the consequences for herself and for others, then it is rarely justifiable to remove her compulsorily. But if her refusal is the result of lack of insight or delusional attitudes to her predicament – that is, if her refusal is itself the result of her mental disorder – removal is probably justified if she cannot reasonably be cared for at home. By this criterion an old lady who is living on her own who has perhaps had several falls or even wandered out into the road but who has a reasonable grasp of her situation and often indicates her wishes forcibly (by some such phrase as "I want to die in my own home") should be left at home, though attempts to persuade her that she needs more care should continue.

If a psychiatrist, balancing the risks against the patient's welfare and civil rights, decides against compulsory admission the general practitioner can reasonably expect him to make his reasons clear in writing and to share the responsibility, for the patient may well come to harm at home or wander out in front of a passing car (the predicament of the motorist who may have her death on his conscience must be considered too). On the other hand, another old person, who is less demented, may insist that she is entirely independent, that she does her own shopping, etc, when she is, in fact, completely dependent on others and virtually confined to one room, and this may justify compulsory admission. But such cases are difficult and always sad. When deciding whether to make a compulsory admission because of the hazards at home weight should also be given to the hazards of an enforced change of surroundings, which is often followed by greater confusion and mysterious decline and death. Clear thinking on these matters demands that the interests of the patient and the interests of other people be distinguished, though each has a right to be considered; errors of both logic and humanity can occur when the one is confused with the other.

No patients (old or young) should ever be denied admission to a medical (or surgical) bed when that is what they need merely because they are under compulsion. Special nursing may have to be provided for such patients in a general ward, but usually they pose few problems. The belief that a confused old person admitted under compulsory powers is likely to be more disturbed than one who has come informally is understandable but false, and it is rarely these patients who upset medical wards.

What supportive services are needed?

An account of the supportive services would make an article in itself, and the unevenness of their availability in different areas is notorious. I list only the main ones; fuller advice should always be available from the area office of the social services department.

(1) Support and surveillance may be sought from social workers, health visitors, district nurses, and, occasionally, specially appointed "geriatric visitors." Community nurses, based either inside or outside the hospital, are an increasingly valuable arm of the services. Some areas offer "family aides."

(2) Home helps and meals on wheels are obtained through the social services department or on direct application to the organiser of the particular service.

(3) Modifications to the home, appliances – such as walking aids or commodes – and disposable incontinence pads or sheets (and in some areas a laundry service) may be arranged through the remedial therapist (often through a home assessment from the hospital), social worker, doctor, or nurse.

(4) Chiropody services are in relatively short supply, as are home physiotherapy and home occupational therapy, which are unobtainable in some areas.

(5) Local authorities may run day centres, often with transport, but these are not always suitable for or willing to receive old people who are behaviourally disturbed: only a minority of areas have special day centres for such people. Many local authorities will accept old people for the day at old people's homes.

(6) In most areas there is a branch of Age Concern, which organises various social activities, such as visiting, clubs, competitions, etc. Other voluntary bodies – for example, MIND – may offer similar help.

(7) The local authority may be able to organise holidays for even quite demented old people.

(8) Most demented old people are so dependent that they qualify for either the full or the partial attendance allowance.

(9) "Relatives' groups," organised by hospital, social services, or voluntary organisations, are helpful to many of those looking after the demented.

(10) The Alzheimer's Disease Society,* a self help organisation for relatives of demented people, has branches in many localities.

* Head office: Bank Buildings, Fulham Broadway, London SW6 1EP. Telephone: 01-381 3177.

Residential accommodation

Residential accommodation is the responsibility of the social services department under part III of the National Assistance Act, and the extent and type of provision vary a great deal up and down the country. Some local authorities have special homes for the "elderly mentally confused," and, though these have been criticised, I believe that properly designed and well run ones are the most appropriate way of meeting the needs of some demented old people. But most demented old people in residential care live in ordinary old people's homes, and dementia itself (as opposed to severe behaviour disorder or dependency on nursing) should not disqualify an old person from a place in such a home. Doctors who are in the habit of visiting old people's homes will already know that it is common for most of the residents to be appreciably demented.

Residential accommodation provided by local authorities is diminishing in relation to the number of very old people who need it. The private sector is expanding rapidly, aided at present by substantial payments from social security (up to £100–200 a week, according to locality) on behalf of residents with capital of less than (at present) £3000. This development of the private sector has been described by Rudolf Klein as "residential care on demand." It raises many urgent issues, notably of quality control (though many homes are excellent) and of the relationship with statutory services.

Sheltered accommodation supervised by wardens is the responsibility of the housing department and is thus administratively separated from residential accommodation. In fact, sheltered accommodation is rarely suitable for a demented old person, unless he or she is to live with a healthy spouse.

Medication

Depression, concurrent illnesses, contributory ailments, and disabilities must, of course, all be treated in their own right. As yet no drugs exist specifically to treat dementia. Drugs that are claimed to improve cerebral blood supply or oxygen utilisation, correct biochemical deficits, or act in other ways are often of theoretical interest but have not yet been proved to be of practical value (and I do not use them). This may yet change in the light of new drugs or convincing evaluations.

The staple drugs in the management of behaviour disturbance in demented old people are the tranquillisers, and there is little evidence that any one is much better than another. It is best to become accustomed to one or two drugs, and I prefer promazine because it is not as potent weight for weight as the other phenothiazines and dosage can thus be more exactly adjusted. When a heavier dosage is required I use thioridazine, chlorpromazine (though this carries a not negligible risk of jaundice), or the butyrophenone haloperidol, which is less sedative and less likely to cause hypotension but more readily causes dystonic effects. Chlormethiazole is useful as a tranquilliser as well as a hypnotic, but a few old people tolerate it poorly, having protracted "hangovers" even though its half life is short. Old people often prefer medicine in liquid form, and syrup is sometimes acceptable when tablets are not. Liquid is harder to hide in the mouth and spit out later than tablets and cannot be hoarded in pockets or under pillows.

Tranquillising regimens should be planned and titrated against the patient's needs. So used they can be an important part of the management not only of confusion but also of paranoid phenomena and of the repetitive questioning and overactivity that can drive relatives to distraction. Shutting the stable door after the horse has bolted – that is, giving large doses when the grossly disturbed behaviour has already occurred – is pointless. In such circumstances the patient is likely simply to become unconscious or possibly even more confused. The aim should be to forestall the disturbance without making the patient dopey. This means taking a careful history of the pattern and circumstances in which the disturbed behaviour most often occurs.

A common problem is nocturnal restlessness, and an increased dose of the tranquillising drug at bedtime together with a hypnotic, such as chloral, will often give a night's sleep to both the patient and her relatives. We make little use of benzodiazepines, but lormetazepam can be useful for some patients, and temazepam, which has a short half life, is favoured by many. These days it is customary not to use barbiturates as hypnotics as in confused old people they may either increase confusion or produce excitement.

Depot tranquillisers in oily solution have only a limited role. The trouble with these drugs, which need to be given only once every three or four weeks (and in old people in half or less the dose for younger people and if necessary more frequently), is that they have a high incidence of dystonic and depressant side effects. Once the injection has been given the effect cannot be wholly reversed until the drugs have been metabolised. Old people with extrapyramidal disease or particularly decrepit old people are unlikely to tolerate these drugs. When a tranquillising regimen is associated with parkinsonian side effects an anti-parkinsonian drug, such as procyclidine 5 mg thrice daily, is given concurrently, though such anticholinergic drugs, notably benzhexol, are themselves prone to causing confusion in old people. When it cannot be controlled by general measures or oral drugs confusional restlessness or excitement almost always responds to intramuscular injection of chlorpromazine 50 mg (or exceptionally 100 mg) or haloperidol 2.5–5 mg.

Tranquillising or antidepressant regimens that are too heavy may make a confused patient more confused. Drug regimens must be reviewed often, and reducing the drugs may be more effective than adding to them. Vitamins have no proved value in dementia unless there is evidence of a deficiency state, but it makes sense to give them to old people who have been living alone and not eating well.

Other practical measures

Problems arising from wandering or incontinence have no easy answers. Control of night time restlessness with drugs may fortify the family by ensuring a night's sleep for everyone. But simple practical measures may go a long way: fitting a lock on a door may stop the old person wandering aimlessly into the street, enabling the family to leave her alone temporarily; a change from more dangerous gas or oil to safer electric appliances can diminish obvious dangers; an approach by the doctor or social worker to a friend or local teenager, whom the family may be shy to ask, may give regular periods of relief when relatives can go shopping or have an evening out. Faecal incontinence is usually due to a remediable cause, such as diarrhoea or impaction, and periodic enemas may solve the problem. Urinary incontinence is dealt with in another chapter.

Conclusion

Old people with failing brains have three main needs: security because their capacity to function physically far outstrips their capacity to adapt to change; stimulation because dementia, especially when accompanied by restricted mobility and sensory privation in the form of deafness or blindness, makes the world a frightening and lonely place, in which withdrawal and apathy may be the way of least resistance; and patience because old people are slow, but time and again they astonish one by their capacity to "get there in the end." Indeed, they are often "there" from the start, and it is their attendants who are too hurried to get there with them.

Of course, these needs are not confined to the demented elderly. They are among the basic needs of all of us, but the disabilities of the demented make their needs more urgent, and their lack of inhibition may make more direct the efforts to satisfy them. The attention seeking behaviour of old people, their wandering and incontinence, may become at least partly intelligible, and so perhaps more manageable, if seen against the background of these needs. But no amount of understanding can make the care of demented old people easy, and the doctor and social worker must beware of attempting to "interpret away" the heavy realities of caring for these severely disabled old people. I hope that this review will be of some practical help but I would not disagree with the view that not all human problems have their solutions.

Further reading

Levy R, Post F, eds. *Psychiatry of late life*. Oxford: Blackwell Scientific Publications, 1982. This textbook contains two chapters on organisation of services, one by Arie and Jolley and one by Hemsi, as well as much other relevant material.

Mace N, Rabins P. *The 36-hour day*. Baltimore: Johns Hopkins Press, 1982. Probably the best guide to dementia for carers.

Arie T, ed. *Recent advances in psychogeriatrics 1*. Edinburgh: Churchill-Livingstone (in press). Contains much material on progress in the dementias.

Drug treatment in the elderly

M R P HALL

Physiological and biochemical changes in aging

Aging is accompanied by many physiological and biochemical changes so that body composition alters and the efficiency of individual organs diminishes – for instance, lean body mass is reduced so that fat mass is relatively increased. Organ blood flow may be diminished, which will result in reduction in the glomerular filtration rate, impairment of renal function, and, consequently, alteration in body salt and water content. Similarly, hepatic metabolism may be less efficient and end organ responses affected. Changes in the composition of cell membrane may alter receptor function, the numbers of receptors on protein molecules may diminish, and nutritional deficiency may lower plasma protein and albumin concentrations.

All these factors will affect the ability of older people to maintain homeostasis, and their response to drugs will differ from that of younger people. How they respond to a particular drug will depend on how that drug is metabolised, which, in turn, will depend on its composition. For instance, many drugs are formulated as bases. Many elderly people eat a protein deficient diet, so that they excrete an acid urine and tend to conserve base: as a result, alkaline drugs will also be conserved and persist for longer in the circulation. Thus pharmacokinetics and pharmacodynamics may be altered, and we should know if this happens. Our knowledge has increased considerably during the past 10 years: nevertheless, iatrogenic disease linked to drugs is very common, and a recent study has shown that it increases in direct relation to the number of drugs being taken.[1] Disease(s) may also adversely affect the metabolism of drugs. A drug, once prescribed, has to be taken, absorbed, metabolised in the liver, transported to the end organ, utilised, and excreted. The steps in this sequence depend on compliance, absorption, hepatic metabolism, transportation by the plasma, distribution in the tissue, and the sensitivity and execution of the organs. Aging may affect each of these steps.

Compliance – The more drugs an old person has to take the worse compliance is likely to be. The maximum number of different preparations that can be managed is probably three, and even then studies suggest that compliance of the third drug will be of the order of 50%. Other factors, particularly those associated with mental impairment, may adversely affect compliance.

Absorption is affected little by aging itself but it may be influenced by the action of other drugs. Laxatives, for example, may speed up the rate of gastrointestinal passage so that absorption of the drug is reduced: on the other hand, some drugs – for example, anticholinergics – may slow down the rate of passage so that absorption is increased. Drugs may interact to form complexes that are less absorbable – for example, tetracycline and iron form a less soluble chelate.[2]

Hepatic metabolism – Various hepatic enzyme systems control drug metabolism and detoxication. Some evidence suggests that the oxidative enzyme process, cytochrome *p*-450 oxidase, is reduced in old age and, therefore, less effective. Another possibility, which has been shown in animals, is that hepatic enzyme induction may be delayed with the effect that drugs reach the systemic circulation without undergoing first pass metabolism[3]: higher concentrations of the drug in the blood might result. Alterations in hepatic blood flow may have the same effect.[4]

Plasma transport – Age reduces the binding sites on plasma protein molecules, particularly albumin. Consequently, more free drug will be available in the case of drugs that are highly protein bound – for example, warfarin or sulphonylureas. The effect, however, is likely to be transitory and will be negated once steady state has occurred. Nevertheless, the possibility of adverse interactions between highly protein bound drugs should be remembered.

Distribution in tissue – Changes in lean and fat body mass and body water lead to changes in distribution of a drug. As a result lipid soluble drugs will have a larger distribution volume and, therefore, a lower plasma concentration, while polar drugs will have a small distribution volume and a high plasma concentration.

Sensitivity of end organs – A considerable quantity of evidence exists that end organ sensitivity increases with age, and this seems particularly to affect the nervous system.[5,6] This may not, however, apply to all end organs, and more research is needed in this field.

Excretion – The glomerular filtration rate diminishes partly because of the reduction of renal blood flow and the number of glomeruli: tubular reabsorption is altered also. The sum effect is that less of the drugs are excreted along with other waste products.

Consequently, the half life is prolonged in the case of drugs that depend on renal excretion to eliminate them and their metabolites.

General principles of drug treatment

When an elderly person does not respond to an effective drug it is nearly always because the patient has failed to take the drug rather than to absorb it. Loading doses of drugs are, therefore, rarely necessary, and in most cases it is better to start with a small dose, particularly if the drug is potentially toxic and likely to be poorly excreted. Large doses of certain drugs should, of course, be given if indicated – for example, antibiotics in acute infections or diuretics in the early stages of heart failure. Nevertheless, in using drugs in the elderly it is wise to observe a few simple rules.

(1) Know the pharmacological action of the drug and, in particular, how it is metabolised and excreted.

(2) Use the lowest dose that is effective in the individual patient. Higher blood concentrations per dose are achieved in the elderly, and the half life of some drugs – for example, cortisol or digoxin – is prolonged. This can lead to accumulation and the need for lower and less frequent doses. Doses should be titrated with patient response, and drug "holidays" may be necessary.

(3) Use as few drugs as possible to meet the needs of the patient. Memory, particularly short term memory, deteriorates with age, and complex drug regimens may not be properly followed. Adverse drug reactions, as well as interactions, are common when many drugs are taken.

(4) Investigate the cause of symptoms before using drugs to treat them. They may be due to social deprivation, which may be better dealt with by a trained social worker.

(5) Do not withhold drugs on account of old age, particularly when drug treatment may improve the old person's quality of life.

(6) Do not use a drug if its side effects are worse than the symptoms it is supposed to relieve. You should know what the side effects of a drug are and remember that adverse reactions may be individual to the patient and may occur with a drug that the patient has taken successfully for many years.

(7) Do not continue to use a drug if it is no longer necessary. It is a wise rule to review repeat prescriptions quarterly in all elderly patients.

(8) Check the patient's self treatment and ensure that it does not affect yours.

Drugs acting on the cardiovascular system

Heart failure is common in old age, and digitalis glycosides remain the key to successful treatment. Their poor tolerance and adverse effects have been known for years. Use of the pure glycoside rather than a preparation of crude digitalis leaf and modern manufacturing techniques may possibly have contributed to this intolerance. Ewy *et al* found that in the elderly the same dose of digoxin produced higher blood concentrations and longer half life.[7] Rules (1) and (2) (see above) apply in the administration of all digitalis derivatives, and great care must be taken: the dose should always be titrated against patient response. An initial dose of 0.5 mg followed by a maintenance dose of 0.125 mg daily is often effective, particularly in the older subject. Occasionally, some individuals need less, in which case the small paediatric/geriatric (PG) tablets of 0.0625 mg strength are useful. Maintenance treatment is probably unnecessary in about 70% of patients,[8] and the drug may be withdrawn quite safely, particularly in those taking 0.0625 mg as a daily maintenance dose.[9]

Potassium depletion is a well known cause of intolerance to digitalis. It results not only from the use of powerful diuretics but may pre-exist due to a reduction in intake of potassium because of poor diet. Serum potassium concentration may be a poor guide to the total body potassium load, though low serum concentrations are nearly always associated with low total body levels.[5,10] Negative potassium balance in congestive heart failure may be high, and large potassium supplements – for example, a minimum of 48 mmol/24 h – are necessary when treating acute heart failure, particularly if diuretics are also used. Nevertheless, as impairment of renal function occurs with age it may not be necessary to give large doses for long, and estimations of blood potassium concentrations should be carried out at weekly intervals until the heart failure is controlled. Once heart failure is controlled, continued maintenance treatment with potassium salts may be unnecessary.[11] If potassium supplements are stopped the patient must be watched for signs of hypokalaemia – namely, confusion, lassitude, anorexia, cardia arrhythmia, and muscular weakness – and blood concentrations should be checked at regular intervals, particularly if diuretics are continued.

Diuretics

Diuretics are commonly used in old people to treat heart failure and oedema. Indeed, they are probably overused to treat dependent oedema, which is unlikely to respond, so that they produce sodium and potassium depletion, postural hypotension, immobility, constipation, and faecal impaction with double incontinence, a state of misery and social inacceptability. Calcium and magnesium depletion may also occur and add to the symptomatology.[12] The actual drug used is a matter of personal choice, as most are effective, but a thiazide diuretic is probably best to use in maintenance and a loop diuretic in the acute phase of treatment. High doses – for example, frusemide 240 mg – may be necessary on occasions. It should be remembered that all diuretics may provoke gout and carbohydrate intolerance. Aldosterone antagonists, such as spironolactone, may potentiate their action and prevent excessive potassium depletion. Dall *et al* have reported that amiloride in combination with hydrochlorothiazide may conserve potassium.[13] Amiloride, however, should be used with caution in the elderly as it may give rise to high blood potassium concentrations.

β Blockers

The β adrenoceptor blocking agents may be used to control angina and supraventricular arrhythmias and to treat hypertension, either alone or in combination with diuretics. Many β blockers are available, and all are effective. They all have similar side effects and will produce bradycardia, precipitate heart failure, and cause cold extremities and bronchospasm, thereby provoking asthma. They may be particularly useful in controlling the tachycardia associated with hyperthyroidism. Which β blocker to use in the elderly is, again, largely a matter of personal preference. If the patient is asthmatic a preparation that is more cardioselective – for example, atenolol or metoprolol – may be preferable. On the other hand a preparation that is water soluble – for example, sotalol or atenolol – has a shorter half life than a lipid soluble preparation and is less likely to give rise to nightmares and sleep disturbance, while a preparation with intrinsic sympathomimetic activity – for example, oxprenolol or pindolol – may cause less bradycardia and coldness of extremities. Nevertheless, propranolol is probably used most widely and seems to give rise to little trouble. Most of these drugs are now available as long acting preparations, thereby helping to simplify drug regimens and improve compliance.

There is little evidence that treating benign hypertension benefits patients over 75 unless they have symptoms, heart failure, or have suffered a stroke. Hypotensive drugs should be used carefully in the elderly and limited to β blockers, diuretics, nifedipine, and, if these are ineffective hydralazine. Verapamil may also be useful, remembering that an interaction may occur between it and β blockers. Nevertheless, rule (5) (see above) applies to hypotensive drugs – that is, use them if their use will enable the patient to lead a more pleasant and active life. Some preparations are likely to produce mental depression, which must be recognised. Similarly, the risk of orthostatic hypotension, with resultant falls and trauma, must be weighed.

Vasodilator drugs

Vasodilator drugs have a place in the treatment of angina and heart failure. Glyceryl trinitrate, which is probably still the most popular, is now available as a spray and a transepidermal preparation as well as in the traditional sublingual form. Long acting forms are available too, and other nitrates – namely, isosorbide dinitrate and isosorbide mononitrate – are also effective. Recognition of the value of vasodilators in treating heart failure is a recent development. Vasodilators act either on the venous side (nitrates) or at the arteriolar site (captopril, hydralazine), or on both sides (prazosin). Peripheral and cerebral vasodilators can no longer be said to have a place in the treatment of the elderly and should not be used.

Drugs acting on the central nervous system

Elderly people commonly suffer from agitation, restlessness, and insomnia. In a busy clinic it can be difficult to elucidate the cause of these symptoms, and thus drugs are often prescribed. Rule (4) particularly applies here, for all drugs acting on the central nervous system are potentially dangerous to the elderly. Nevertheless, they may be effective in relieving symptoms and, hence, useful. Some old people are extremely sensitive to certain of these drugs[6,7]; even quite small doses may produce soporific states, and, therefore small doses should be used initially.

Of the hypnotics, chlormethiazole (Heminevrin) is probably the most useful as it has a short half life and does not produce long term sedation. Modern chloral derivatives, such as dichloralphenazone (Welldorm) or triclofos (Tricloryl), are also possibilities, and so are short acting benzodiazepines such as temazepam and lormetazepam. Rule (7) applies to all these drugs, and they should be stopped as soon as possible. Barbiturates are not recommended because the elderly tolerate them poorly and they may give rise to lethargy, depression, and confusion.

Sedatives and tranquillisers

Of the sedatives and tranquillisers, diazepam (Valium) and chlordiazepoxide (Librium) are the most widely used. Both drugs, however, may provoke a feeling of weakness in some old people, particularly patients who have had cerebrovascular accidents. Agitation and hallucinations are most easily controlled by drugs from the phenothiazine group. Despite its tendency to give rise to jaundice in some people, chlorpromazine (Largactil) is probably the most effective and widely used. Doses should be kept as small as possible, starting preferably with 10 mg, and increasing this as necessary. Promazine (Sparine), which is weaker, and thioridazine (Melleril), which may be more effective in some patients, are alternatives to chlorpromazine. More potent drugs in this group are trifluoperazine (Stelazine) and haloperidol (Serenace), which comes in the form of colourless and tasteless drops and may be particularly useful in controlling highly agitated patients. A small dose of 0.5–1.5 mg thrice daily is often sufficient. Similarly, the decanoate and enanthate forms of fluphenazine may be useful as a single injection will control symptoms for quite long periods. It should be remembered that all these drugs produce side effects and, in particular, may unmask features of parkinsonism so that antiparkinsonian preparations may have to be given simultaneously. In addition, these drugs should not be used in patients vulnerable to accidental hypothermia; they may also provoke postural hypotension.

The incidence of depressive illness rises with age, and a psychiatrist should supervise the treatment of patients with this condition. Short courses of electroshock therapy may often be more effective than the taking of drugs for long periods. If drugs are used the tricyclic group of antidepressant drugs is most useful. These drugs may cause urinary retention, constipation, and the precipitation or aggravation of glaucoma. They may also provoke severe postural hypotension and aggravate dryness of the mouth, even causing lingual or oral ulcers. Rules (1) and (2) apply particularly to the use of all these drugs, although large doses should not be withheld from patients who need them.

Parkinson's disease

Treatment of Parkinson's disease with levodopa represents a considerable advance, but it must be used carefully because failure of treatment is often due to incorrect prescription. The initial dose may be as low as 62.5 mg daily, and increments may be at weekly intervals until the daily dose equals 0.5–1.0 g. Some elderly patients respond to amantadine hydrochloride in an initial dose of 100 mg daily, which is increased to 100 mg twice daily after one week. This may, however, give rise to confusional states and is probably ineffective after about three months. Severe nausea and vomiting are common adverse reactions to levodopa, which may be due to peaking of blood concentrations: the addition of a dopa decarboxylase inhibitor can prevent this happening. The optimum dose of levodopa may be found to be lower than in younger patients, and improvement may continue for months or even years. The older antiparkinsonian drugs may have a place in the treatment of patients who cannot tolerate L-dopa, but they should all be used with care, and rules (1) and (2) apply. Other newer drugs are bromocriptine and selegiline, both of which may be useful in helping to control symptoms and improve function if levodopa fails.

Relief of pain

Pain and discomfort are common symptoms, being associated with skeletal disorders as well as with cancer.[14-16] Preventing pain is, without doubt, much easier than relieving it once it has occurred. Pain should not be allowed to ebb and flow; if analgesics, sedatives, anti-inflammatory drugs, and narcotics are given regularly and patients are instructed in their proper use pain can be prevented from developing and symptoms minimised as much as possible.

Soluble aspirin remains probably the most effective analgesic, particularly in the treatment of skeletal, as opposed to visceral, pain. The possibility of gastrointestinal bleeding must be remembered: some preparations – for example, Benorylate, Safapryn, or Caprin – may be safer but are more expensive. Paracetamol, either alone or combined with other analgesics, is safer but less effective, although, by enhancing its absorption, sorbitol may improve its action. The anti-inflammatory drugs phenylbutazone (Butazolidin), indomethacin (Indocid), and ibuprofen (Brufen) can relieve pain effectively, and so can other non-steroidal anti-inflammatory drugs (NSAIDs), but all these tend to give rise to gastrointestinal symptoms. In cases of severe pain small doses of narcotics may be used if given in conjunction with chlorpromazine, enabling the patient to remain alert yet free from pain. New formulations may be useful – for example, sublingual buprenorphine or meptazinol, which is effective and non-cumulative in the elderly.[17] In cases of very severe pain diamorphine remains the preferred drug, given in combination with chlorpromazine.

Corticosteroids rarely need to be used and should be avoided unless specifically indicated. They are sometimes useful in treating arthralgia that has not responded to other analgesics, when intra-articular injections may afford considerable relief. In widespread arthralgia – for example, late onset rheumatoid arthritis – large doses may be necessary but should be reduced as soon as symptoms are controlled. Large doses may also be needed in the treatment of asthma and in the treatment of temporal arteritis and polymyalgia rheumatica, when the initial dose should be high and reduction, which should be achieved as rapidly as possible, titrated against the erythrocyte sedimentation rate. All patients should undergo chest radiography to exclude pulmonary tuberculosis, which may be reactivated by steroid treatment.

Treatment of infection

Antibacterial drugs have no special contraindications in the elderly. It should, however, be remembered that many are poorly eliminated: thus blood concentrations will be higher and toxic reactions may be more common. Streptomycin and gentamicin should be used with care, and blood concentrations should be monitored. Antibiotic and antibacterial drugs should be given by mouth as injections may cause sterile abscesses, and the resulting tissue breakdown may produce pressure sores. Concomitant monilial infections may occur in patients who are severely debilitated.

Conclusions

In a short article it is impossible to cover all aspects of drug treatment in the elderly. Other forms of treatment include hormone replacement therapy, using hormones such as thyroxine, or treatment with vitamins, such as vitamin B_{12} and folic acid. Vitamins, particularly C and D, and minerals, such as iron, may be indicated in housebound and other elderly patients prone to subnutrition. Though no preparations exist that will specifically combat old age, the elderly will benefit as much from appropriate drug treatment as any young person. The key to good drug treatment is accurate diagnosis, assessment of the objectives of treatment, and use of the appropriate drug or drugs, bearing in mind the rules already outlined that should govern the use of any drug. Good treatment with drugs is not easy but it is rewarding.

[1] Williamson J, Chopin JM. Adverse reactions to prescribed drugs in the elderly: A multicentre investigation. *Age Ageing* 1980; **9**: 73–81.
[2] Stockley IH. *Drug interactions.* Oxford: Blackwell Scientific Publications, 1981: 106.
[3] Adelman RC. *Age dependent control of enzyme adaption in advances in gerontological research.* Strehler B, ed. New York and London: Academic Press, 1972: 1–23.
[4] Castleden CM, George CF. The effect of ageing on the hepatic clearance of propranolol. *Br J Clin Pharmacol* 1979; **7**: 49–54.
[5] Evans JG, Jarvis EH. Nitrazepam in old age. *Br Med J* 1972; **iv**: 487.
[6] Castleden CM, George CF, Marcer D, Hallett C. Increased sensitivity to nitrazepam in old age. *Br Med J* 1977; **i**: 10–12.

⁷ Ewy GA, Kapadia GG, Yao L, Lullin M, Marcus FI. Digoxin metabolism in the elderly. *Circulation* 1969; **39**: 449–53.

⁸ Dall JLC. Maintenance digoxin in elderly patients. *Br Med J* 1970, ii: 705–6.

⁹ Bansal A, Hall MRP. The importance of calcium/potassium interaction in digoxin toxicity. *Journal of Clinical and Experimental Gerontology* 1982; **4**: 307–26.

¹⁰ Cox JR, Pearson RD, Speight CJ. Changes in sodium, potassium and body fluid spaces in depression and dementia. *Gerontologia clinica* 1971; **13**: 233–45.

¹¹ Down PF, Polak A, Rao R, Mead JA. Fate of potassium supplements in 6 outpatients receiving long-term diuretics for oedematous disease. *Lancet* 1972; ii: 721.

¹² Thomas AJ, Hodkinson HM. Which diuretics cause hypomagnesaemia? *Journal of Clinical and Experimental Gerontology* 1981; **3**: 269–84.

¹³ Dall JLC, MacFarland JPR, Kennedy RD. Dangers of diuretic therapy in elderly patients. In: Steinmann B, ed. *Proceedings of the VIth European congress of clinical gerontology*. Berne: Huber, 1971: 371–3.

¹⁴ Sinclair D. The Anatomy and physiology of pain. *Br J Hosp Med* 1973; **9**: 568–71.

¹⁵ Merskey H. The management of patients in pain. *Br J Hosp Med* 1973; **9**: 574–80.

¹⁶ Lipton S. The medical treatment of pain. *Br J Hosp Med* 1973; **9**: 583–6.

¹⁷ Norbury HM, Franklin RA, Graham DS, Sinha B. Pharmacokinetics of meptazinol after single and multiple oral administration to elderly patients. *Eur J Clin Pharmacol*. (in press).

Gastrointestinal problems in the old: symptoms

DENNIS E HYAMS, PETER J ROYLANCE

Gastrointestinal symptoms and diseases increase with aging. The most common lesions are carcinoma (of the stomach or large bowel), peptic ulceration, intestinal obstruction (hernia or diverticular disease of the colon), hiatus hernia, and gall stones. The first three of these caused most of the 20% of deaths directly due to lesions of the digestive system reported by McKeown in her study of a series of 1500 necropsies in patients aged 70 or over.[1] This incidence was second only to that of deaths caused by diseases of the cardiovascular system and, numerically, only a little less. Carcinomas of the gastrointestinal system constituted nearly half of all fatal malignant disease, and half of these carcinomas were in the large bowel. It has been reported that disease of the biliary tract is the most common condition that requires abdominal surgery in the aged.[2] In elderly patients with abdominal pain Ponka et al found that disease of the gall bladder was the cause in 27.5%.[3]

Whether functional changes in the gut contribute greatly to gastrointestinal morbidity in old age is doubtful. Nevertheless, changes have been described in the following functions: the flow and composition of saliva, gastric juice, bile, and pancreatic juice; the motility of the stomach and large bowel; absorption from the small intestine; and flora of the large bowel. Associated structural changes have also been described.[4]

Anorexia

Reduction in appetite may arise because of impaired sense of smell and taste, limited activity, dull food, psychological reasons, or because of various organic disease states. About 10% of old people are housebound, which increases their vulnerability to many problems. When physical disabilities, lack of help, or mental confusion make it hard for old people to shop their food may be dull or inadequate. Depression, isolation, loneliness, apathy, and negativism are all well known causes of anorexia in the elderly, who are especially vulnerable after bereavement, more so if living alone. Anorexia is seen in disease of the digestive system, notably carcinoma of the stomach, but it is also a common symptom in physical disorders elsewhere that have secondary effects on the stomach, such as heart failure, anaemia, and uraemia, and anorexia may also arise from their treatment – for example, with digitalis (see below).

Management

Underlying causes must be identified and dealt with. Food should be attractively presented. Attempts to stimulate a poor appetite in old people by drugs, such as cyproheptadine, the old fashioned nux vomica, or "tonics," such as Villescon, are rarely successful, but alcohol may be more useful. Supplementary feeding – for example, with Complan – may be necessary to sustain the patient over a difficult period in or after an acute illness: in a very weak or ill patient feeding may have to be by gastric tube, and, rarely, parenteral feeding is required. Some very old people reject food or spit it out during feeding. In such cases tube feeding should be started only after considering carefully medical and ethical aspects of the problem. Nevertheless, even in these cases it is important to avoid dehydration.

Increased appetite in the elderly is usually psychogenic. It is rarely a feature in the elderly thyrotoxic patient.

Nausea and vomiting

Nausea and vomiting may arise not only in diseases of the digestive system itself but also in diseases located primarily elsewhere, which warrant consideration in more detail. Thus heart failure leads to gastric congestion and may produce anorexia, nausea, and vomiting. Cardiac infarction may also be associated with these symptoms. Courses of drug treatment in normal recommended adult doses may cause nausea and vomiting. Morphine and pethidine are generally considered to be two of the most potent emetic compounds in clinical use, and response to these drugs in the elderly, as in other age groups, varies widely. Non-steroidal anti-inflammatory drugs in normal therapeutic doses provoke nausea and vomiting in some elderly patients. Other drugs, particularly when given in relative overdose, may produce vomiting – for example, in digitalis intoxication – although in the old, this is more likely to present as an arrhythmia or a confusional state, which is an important cause of morbidity in the elderly. Plasma digoxin assays may be helpful if correlated with the clinical state, but in all cases digoxin dosage must be related to renal function.

Other drugs may produce nausea and vomiting – for example, oestrogens, codeine, dihydrocodeinone, or metformin. Metabolic disorders are another important cause, especially uraemia, diabetic ketosis, and hypercalcaemia. Labyrinthine disturbance, neurological disorders, and infections are other possible causes. Tumours, radiotherapy, chemotherapy, some inhaled anaesthetics, and raised intracranial pressure are often responsible for nausea and vomiting. In addition, psychogenic stimuli should not be overlooked – for example, fear, anxiety, and the universal stimulus of seeing other patients being sick.

Management

The essential principle in management is to determine and treat the underlying cause. Drug induced nausea and vomiting require reduction in dose or withdrawal of the drug. Antihistamines are time honoured antiemetics but currently are used mainly for travel sickness. Phenothiazine antiemetics act principally on the chemoreceptor trigger zone located in the medulla, adjacent to the vomiting centre. Both these groups of drugs possess sedative and soporific side effects, which may be stronger in the elderly patient, who is often unduly susceptible to such effects. Metoclopramide (Maxolon), a dopamine antagonist, may be of value in the elderly because of its unique actions: it inhibits the chemoreceptor trigger zone, raises pressure at the lower oesophageal sphincter, increases the frequency and amplitude of gastric contractions in synchrony with duodenal contractions, and thus speeds up the passage of stomach contents into and through the small intestine. Side effects, such as lassitude, drowsiness, and extrapyramidal reactions, seem more common in younger people.

Dysphagia

Dysphagia is a common and important complaint in old people. It must never be regarded as functional unless the fullest possible investigation has been carried out, but even then the patient must undergo careful and frequent reviews. The patient may have difficulty in swallowing solids but not liquids, and some types of solid food can be easier to cope with than others. Food may stick consistently at a certain level, then moving on or being regurgitated, but the elderly patient may describe the level inaccurately. At times the initiation of the swallowing reflex seems impaired, and food is chewed for long periods but finally rejected. The risk of

Causes of dysphagia

Type and position	Causes
Local	
Mouth	Tongue lesions, especially carcinoma
Larynx	Carcinoma
Pharynx	Diverticulum (usually traction)
	Postcricoid web (Paterson-Kelly syndrome) or carcinoma
	Infections, abscess
Oesophagus	
Intrinsic	Carcinoma (especially mid level)
	Stricture (hiatus hernia)
	Spasm ("corkscrew" oesophagus)
	Achalasia
Extrinsic	Diverticula (traction)
	Pressure from unfolded aorta (dysphagia lusoria)
Stomach	Foreign body
	Carcinoma of cardia
	Hiatus hernia: rolling (paraoesophageal) or sliding with ulceration or stricture
Remote: neurological	Disorders of the brain stem: pseudobulbar palsy, stroke, posterior inferior cerebellar artery syndrome

"spill-over" into the trachea is common in patients with dysphagia of neurological origin, and they may be afraid to swallow. It should always be remembered that dysphagia is a source of alarm to an elderly patient, for whom it carries the fear of cancer. The table lists the various causes of dysphagia.

Management

The primary cause must be dealt with as effectively as possible. Mechanical obstruction of the oesophagus – for example, carcinoma or stricture – is suggested by dysphagia mainly for solids. Motor dysfunction – for example, achalasia – usually causes dysphagia for liquids as well as solids. Achalasia may be secondary to a neoplasm in the region of the gastro-oesophageal junction: secondary achalasia may be suspected in the elderly patient if the history is short and weight loss rapid. It has been reported that peristaltic activity in the oesophagus becomes impaired in old age,[5,6] and this condition has been termed "presbyoesophagus." But these motor changes rarely lead to clinical symptoms, and this diagnosis is probably best avoided,[7] especially as some authors failed to find any such age related changes.[8,9] Specific treatment may sometimes help – for example, L-dopa in parkinsonism, cholinesterase inhibitors in myasthenia gravis, or corticosteroids in dermatomyositis. Webs may be broken and strictures dilated. Sedatives should be avoided if possible.

Tube feeding

The ethical dilemmas posed by prolonged tube feeding have already been mentioned briefly. The decision whether to tube feed is influenced, on the one hand by the likely prognosis in the patient and her quality of life, and on the other by the likely mode of death, which is an aspect that doctors too often neglect. Neither choking nor dehydration permits death with dignity. If it proves impossible to pass a nasogastric tube a Mousseau-Barbin or Celestin tube may be inserted at oesophagoscopy in order to maintain a lumen. Gastrostomy is not justified in the elderly and perhaps not at any age, as it produces so much distress itself. An excellent review of oesophageal disorders in the elderly has appeared recently.[10]

Change in bowel habit

Changes in bowel habit must always be taken seriously.

Diarrhoea

Acute diarrhoea may occur for the usual reasons (food poisoning, dietary indiscretion), but inquiries should also cover the possibility of an abuse of purgatives. Other drugs may produce diarrhoea as a side effect. Spurious diarrhoea due to faecal impaction (see below) is common in old people. Chronic diarrhoea raises the suspicion of carcinoma of the colon or rectum but it may also be due to other diseases of the gastrointestinal tract, especially diverticular disease of the colon, ulcerative coloproctitis, or faecal impaction, a common cause. Diarrhoea may be due to steatorrhoea, possibly after an earlier partial gastrectomy. Systemic disorders associated with diarrhoea include uraemia, diabetes, thyrotoxicosis, and liver disease. Psychogenic causes may occur in old age, as in younger persons. Old people with diarrhoea may develop faecal incontinence: firstly, because their desire to defecate is too urgent and because their stool is fluid or semi-formed; secondly, because their mobility is possibly impaired and the lavatory may also be too far away; and, thirdly, and only occasionally, because of laxity or weakness of the anal sphincter.

Faecal incontinence

The causes of faecal incontinence may be local or distant. Of local causes, diarrhoea is the most common, but rectal prolapse or prolapsed haemorrhoids may be present. Faecal incontinence is rarely due to simple weakness or laxity of the sphincter. Distant causes include brain damage or dementia, leading to lack of cortical inhibition, but this cause is less common than a local cause (the reverse applies in urinary incontinence). Spinal cord lesions are rare causes of faecal incontinence in the old. Faecal incontinence can be the last straw that breaks down attempts to nurse an old person at home. Moreover, the patient is falsely labelled as "senile" or "mental," which may lead to mistaken placement of the patient in a mental hospital.

Constipation

Many old people are constipated, and even more are convinced that they are, as preoccupation with the bowels is common in old age. Constipation is important because it may lead to severe complications. Rather than thinking of constipation in terms of the time taken by transit through the gut, which is slowed in old age [11,12] without necessarily causing symptoms, it is better to look at the type of faeces produced – that is, whether they are hard and dry. About half the elderly people studied in various surveys take laxatives, often unnecessarily.

Primary causes of constipation are: slow transit time (especially in bedfast patients); incomplete emptying of the bowel because of poor muscle tone, unsatisfactory toilet arrangements, laziness, mental confusion, or dementia; diminished awareness of a loaded or overloaded rectum; neglect of the call to defaecate; a diet low in bulk foods, perhaps due to ignorance, lack of money, or poor dentition; and inadequate fluid, sometimes due to fear of urinary difficulties.

Secondary causes of constipation may be gastrointestinal or otherwise. Diverticular disease of the colon and carcinoma of the colon or rectum must be considered. Anorectal lesions such as fissures, haemorrhoids, or pectenosis [13] may contribute.

Other important causes include: drugs, such as codeine and dihydrocodeine, morphine, iron, aluminium compounds, calcium salts, and anticholinergics; hypothyroidism; and mental disorders. In addition, as is often the case in the elderly, a combination of several factors may be responsible for producing the constipation. The figure by Wilkins illustrates the vicious circles that can develop. [14]

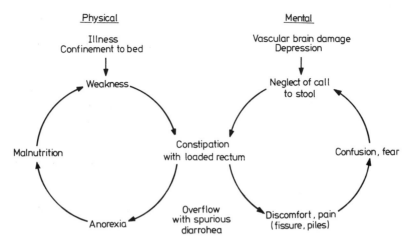

Vicious circles of constipation in the elderly.[14]

The main complication of constipation is faecal impaction. Faecal retention plus absorption of fluid in the large bowel leads to hardening of faeces, which are packed together by peristaltic waves and lubricated by excess secretion of mucus. The impaction over distends the rectum, although occasionally it occurs higher in the colon while the rectum remains empty. Sometimes impaction of a great mass of soft faeces occurs in weak patients. Faecal impaction may lead to the following problems.

Faecal incontinence – Impacted faeces act like a ball valve so that more watery stool at a higher level leaks around the faecal mass. Stretching of the anal ring is corrected only when the rectum is cleared; until then the "spurious diarrhoea" will continue.

Intestinal obstruction – This may have a high mortality or may lead to unnecessary surgical intervention.

Mental disturbances – Restlessness and confusion may be due to faecal impaction: this could be termed the "recto-cephalic reflex." This simple mechanism is worth remembering when dealing with disturbed or restless old people: it could avoid many an unwarranted admission to hospital. Sedation of the patient without a preliminary rectal examination is poor medical practice.

Retention of urine – This may be associated with overflow urinary incontinence, possibly due to pressure of the distended rectum on the neck of the bladder.

Rectal bleeding – This may arise from ulceration of the mucosa: the presence of a neoplasm must be excluded.

Other gastrointestinal effects may occur with constipation – for example, megacolon, with an atonic colon, or volvulus of the colon, producing intestinal obstruction. Gross gaseous distension of the bowel may produce angina pectoris and electrocardiographic changes.

Another important complication of constipation results from straining. Adverse effects of straining have been clearly shown on the coronary, cerebral, and peripheral arterial circulation. In the elderly with cerebrovascular disease transient ischaemic attacks may occur. In patients whose baroreceptor reflexes are impaired and who have a tendency to postural hypotension, straining at stool produces the Valsalva manoeuvre and syncope may develop.[15] This mechanism may account for the common history of finding the patient on the lavatory floor. Symptoms of hiatus hernia may be aggravated by the rise in intra-abdominal pressure on straining.

Management of diarrhoea

Proper management of diarrhoea is impossible without a rectal examination. The treatment must deal with the underlying cause as far as possible. In acute cases demanding symptomatic treatment, food should be withheld for up to 24 hours but fluids given liberally to avoid dehydration. Kaolin or chalk may help in selected cases but they should not be used when combined with opiates unless the cause of diarrhoea has been diagnosed with reasonable certainty. In the elderly these medicines should be used with care: it is bad clinical practice to give kaolin mixtures to patients with diarrhoea that is spurious and secondary to faecal impaction. Injudicious use of opiates may mask the diagnosis of important abdominal disorder. Diphenoxylate (Lomotil) or loperamide (Imodium) help to reduce the time taken for transit through the intestine. Codeine phosphate tablets are useful but may encourage vomiting. Hydrophilic bulking agents, such as methylcellulose, while mainly useful in the treatment of constipation, may also be of value in treating diarrhoea if taken with jam rather than water. They then absorb water from the stool and improve its consistency, which is particularly helpful in regulating the function of a colostomy. Most cases of diarrhoea do not have a bacterial origin. In general, antibiotic and sulphonamide preparations should be withheld in order to avoid the development of bacterial resistance and pseudomembranous enterocolitis. Similar considerations apply to the management of chronic diarrhoea, in which accurate diagnosis is essential, and fluid and electrolyte (especially potassium) balance need particular attention.

Management of constipation

In the management of constipation the underlying causes must also be treated individually. In general management of the problem reassurance and explanation will help if habits need retraining; the extent of physical activity, fluid intake, and the amount of bulk in the diet may require attention. Some old people benefit from a glass of hot water first thing in the morning as a regular habit. Toilet arrangements may require revision. Though low lavatory seats are difficult for the elderly to cope with, some degree of squatting aids defecation, and excessive zeal in raising the level of the seat may actually hinder efficient defecation. Nevertheless, polyethylene seat raisers are helpful to many arthritic old people.

Laxatives fall into three main types. Firstly, there are bulking agents. Many people (old and young) live on diets low in fibre content, which produce small, hard, and infrequent stools. Bulking agents are bland and absorb water, increasing the volume of the stool, and they are the most physiological way of dealing with constipation and diverticular disease of the colon. Unprocessed bran is a useful additive to the diet in such cases (and helps in their prevention): it may be sprinkled on cereals or other foodstuffs. Most old people would probably benefit from consuming bran regularly, but it has a high content of phytic acid, which might impair calcium absorption in subjects with latent or overt vitamin D deficiency, and evidence is increasing to show that this may be commoner in the elderly than previously thought. Some evidence suggests that the texture of bran affects its clinical efficacy and that coarse bran may be advantageous.[16,17] Other hydrophilic agents in this category include semisynthetic cellulose ethers (Celevac and Cologel) and mucilaginous substances (Isogel and Normacol). These agents should be taken with abundant liquids to avoid the potential hazard of intestinal obstruction from bolus formation, especially when intestinal motility is reduced or if intestinal disease is present. The second type of laxative is the stimulant variety. Senna is the best representative of the anthracene laxatives and is available in standardised form as Senokot. It works mainly on the transverse and distal colon, so that while stools are likely to be formed fluid and electrolyte disturbances are unlikely. Bisacodyl (Dulcolax) is a contact laxative and more likely than Senokot to produce liquid stools and, in the elderly, faecal incontinence: it is also more likely to cause severe griping. Phenolphthalein has little place in modern treatment; its effects are more unpredictable than those of senna as it is reabsorbed from the intestine and acts repeatedly. The other stimulant laxatives, including irritants like colocynth, jalap, podophyllum, aloes (all contained in vegetable laxative tablets), and croton oil, have no place in the management of constipation at any age. Thirdly, there are the osmotic laxatives, or "salts" – soluble sulphates, phosphates, or tartrates of sodium, potassium, or magnesium – that act through the osmotic effects of their ions, which results in the retention of large volumes of fluid throughout the bowel. The disturbance to normal gut physiology is considerable: the stools are loose and fluid and electrolyte disturbances likely. These agents are best reserved for special indications only – for example, food poisoning. Lactulose is effective only when acted on by colonic bacteria, but it may have undesirable effects on these bacteria and cause gaseous distension. It may be useful to clear the colon in hepatic failure and where there is colonic retention of barium after a barium meal.[18]

Stool softeners – Dioctyl sodium sulphosuccinate (docusate sodium, DOS) and poloxalkols are surface active "wetting" agents, which are said to penetrate hard stools and help to soften them. While they are being taken they are also said to prevent the formation of hard stools. They are popular in geriatric practice, but the possible effects (especially long term ones) of the consumption of detergents are not yet fully known. In animals they cause changes in gut physiology. Preparations that combine these agents with stimulant laxatives – for example, bisacodyl plus docusate sodium (Dulcodos) or danthron plus poloxalkols (Dorbanex) – have been found useful in geriatric patients, but, again, some caution is advised as other combinations of this type have had adverse effects in large doses or in long term usage. Liquid paraffin, once thought harmless, has now earned itself a bad name. It may impair absorption of fat soluble vitamins, leak from the anus, be aspirated into the lungs to cause lipoid pneumonia, and may be absorbed (especially when given in emulsion form) and deposited in body tissues. These risks are greater in the elderly, and its use should be avoided, at least as a regular habit.

Rectal evacuation – Suppositories of glycerin of bisacodyl are sometimes helpful, although bisacodyl may cause local discomfort. Enemas should be small volume solutions, containing oil for softening and saline for evacuation. Disposable hypertonic saline enemas are convenient, gentle, and reasonably effective. Soap should never be used in enemas.

Manual removal of faeces may be required in the initial treatment of faecal impaction because oral laxatives cannot be expected to clear the bowel when the lower end is plugged so effectively with accumulated faeces. Suppositories and enemas may also fail in these circumstances, although a small volume enema should be tried as the first step. This may be repeated daily and its efficacy tested by repeated digital examinations. With soft faecal impaction bisacodyl suppositories may also be successful: one should be used high up in the rectum and repeated once if nothing has happened after two hours. Large volume washouts with saline may be needed to clear the lower bowel if impaction is high above the rectum.

Management of faecal incontinence

As most cases of faecal incontinence are due to spurious diarrhoea associated with faecal impaction treatment of the impaction will deal with the incontinence. For the neurogenic type of faecal incontinence a regimen of kaolin and morphine mixture 15 ml every morning, alternating with Senokot one to two tablets every night, has been advocated by Jarrett and Exton-Smith.[19] In such cases it is essential to exclude the presence of faecal impaction.

1 McKeown F. *Pathology of the aged*. London: Butterworth, 1965.
2 Strohl EL, Diffenbaugh WG, Anderson RE. Biliary tract surgery in the aged patient. *Geriatrics* 1964; **19**: 275–9.
3 Ponka JL, Welborn JK, Brush BE. Acute abdominal pain in aged patients: an analysis of 200 cases. *J Am Geriatr Soc* 1963; **11**: 993–1007.
4 Hyams DE. Nutrition of the elderly. *Modern Geriatrics* 1973; **3**: 352.
5 Khan TA, Shragge BW, Crispin JS, Lind JF. Esophageal motility in the elderly. *Am J Dig Dis* 1977; **22**: 1049–54.
6 Csendes A, Guiraldes E, Bancalari A, Braghetto I, Ayala M. Relation of gastroesophageal sphincter pressure and serum gastrin studies following food intake before and after vagotomy for duodenal ulcer. *Scan J Gastroenterol* 1973; **13**: 443–7.
7 Altman DF. Gastrointestinal diseases in the elderly. *Med Clin North Am* 1983; **67**: 433–4.
8 Hollis JB, Castell DO. Esophageal function in elderly men. A new look at "presbyesophagus." *Ann Intern Med* 1974; **80**: 371.
9 Hollis JB, Castell DO. Effect of dry swallows and wet swallows of different volumes on esophageal peristalsis. *J Appl Physiol* 1975; **38**: 1161–4.
10 Hellemans J, Vantrappen G, Pelemans W. Oesophageal disorders in old people. In: Isaacs B, ed. *Recent advances in geriatric medicine 2*. London: Churchill Livingstone, 1982: 91.
11 Hyams DE. The absorption of vitamin B$_{12}$ in the elderly. *Gerontologia Clinica* 1964; **6**: 193–206.
12 Brocklehurst JC, Kahn MV. A study of faecal stasis in old age and the use of "dorbanex" in its prevention. *Gerontologia Clinica* 1969; **11**: 293–300.
13 Exton-Smith AN. Constipation in geriatrics. In: Jones AF, Godding EW, eds. *Management of constipation*. Oxford: Blackwell Scientific Publications, 1972: 156–75.
14 Wilkins EG. Constipation in the elderly. *Postgrad Med J* 1968; **44**: 728–32.
15 Pathy MS. Defaecation syncope. *Age Ageing* 1978; **7**: 233–6.
16 Smith AN, Drummond E, Eastwood MA. The effect of coarse and fine Canadian red spring wheat and french soft wheat bran on colonic motility in patients with diverticular disease. *Am J Clin Nutr* 1981; **34**: 2460–3.
17 Pringle R, Pennington MJ, Pennington CR, Ritchie RT. A study of the influence of a fibre biscuit on bowel function in the elderly. *Age Ageing* 1984; **13**: 175–8.

[18] Prout BJ, Datta SB, Wilson TS. Colonic retention of barium in the elderly after barium-meal examination and its treatment with lactulose. *Br Med J* 1972; iv: 530–3.

[19] Jarrett AS, Exton-Smith AN. Treatment of faecal incontinence. *Lancet* 1960, i: 925.

Gastrointestinal problems in the old: causes

DENNIS E HYAMS, PETER J ROYLANCE

Acute abdomen

The acute abdomen often causes considerable problems in elderly patients.[1] Its presentation may be atypical, and the later the diagnosis is made, the more stormy the course and the more likely complications will be, especially at and after surgery.

Often old people cannot cope as well as younger patients with their illness so that early diagnosis becomes of major importance. Yet these are often the very patients who are diagnosed late because of difficulties in communication, few or atypical symptoms, absence of "classical" physical signs, and problems in physical examination due to associated degenerative or disease processes. Pain may be absent or unimpressive, and the description of its type and site is often vague. Abdominal rigidity and even guarding may be absent, which would certainly have been present in earlier years. In such patients the presence or absence of gut sounds can be a most important physical sign as the condition is, in many ways, analogous to the acute abdomen that develops in patients being treated with steroids.

Complications occur frequently – for example, complications of acute appendicitis are found at operation five times more often in old than in younger patients. Peritonitis from whatever cause is kept localised less effectively in elderly patients. The mortality of major operations in the elderly is considerably higher, especially if the operation is performed as an emergency, and it increases as age advances.

A good general rule to follow is that elderly people with severe abdominal pain should be admitted to hospital even if they show no physical signs. The elderly have many medical causes of acute abdominal pain, including acute pancreatitis, diabetic ketosis, tabes dorsalis, Addison's disease, hypercalcaemia, haemochromatosis, or porphyria. Vascular bowel diseases have become better recognised (see below); acute mesenteric vascular occlusion and ischaemic colitis may produce an acute abdomen. Furthermore, abdominal pain may be due to extra-abdominal diseases, such as pleurisy, spondylosis, zoster, etc, which are common in old people.

Diverticular disease

Small intestine – Duodenal diverticula are common, being second in prevalence only to colonic diverticula and occurring in about 10% of people over the age of 55. They were regarded for a long time as being of little or no clinical importance unless complications developed, but in a review of the literature in 1972, in which he also reported 15 new cases, Clark emphasised that duodenal diverticular disease may be associated with alterations in bowel flora, producing a form of stagnant loop syndrome with malabsorption and deficiency states analogous to those found in jejunal diverticulosis.[2] The deficiencies in duodenal diverticular disease seem to differ in prevalence from those in jejunal diverticulosis in that iron, folate, and vitamin B_{12} deficiency were seen in that order of frequency, the reverse of the jejunal pattern. This may be because the alterations in bowel flora in duodenal cases are localised to the upper small intestine.

Colon – Colonic diverticula develop in middle and later life, especially in the obese and the constipated. They occur in one in three people over 60 and in more than one in two of those in their 80s and 90s.[3] The diverticula result from a disturbance of colonic motility, which is often due to hypertrophy of the smooth muscle, tending to produce high intraluminal pressures in the colon. Diets that are deficient in fibre are associated with long intestinal transit times and small infrequent stools. Such diets, with their abundance of refined carbohydrate, encouraging fermentation in the intestine, also lead to abnormal increases of pressure in the bowel and are important factors in the pathogenesis of diverticulosis coli.[4] It is difficult to differentiate diverticulosis from diverticulitis clinically and often radiologically.[5] Three clinical patterns may be recognised. Firstly, most cases are asymptomatic. Secondly, symptoms may arise in uncomplicated cases and consist of abdominal discomfort, pain in the left iliac fossa, and constipation or diarrhoea. Thirdly, in complicated diverticular disease pain, tenderness, fever, and bleeding per rectum may occur. In some cases a mass may also be evident in the left side of the abdomen and occasionally the bladder is affected. In addition, a pericolic abscess may form and perforate. It is worth remembering that diverticular disease of the colon has been called "the great imitator."

Treatment has traditionally been with a low residue diet, but

Painter showed that unprocessed bran was effective in relieving symptoms.[6] Unprocessed bran is cheap and easily taken: daily doses of 2–12 g (one to six teaspoonfuls) have been recommended, which should be continued throughout life, even in asymptomatic cases, except when complications are present. Coarser forms of bran may be even better. Acute symptoms also call for a low residue diet, and drugs may also be required – for example, antibiotics if infection is diagnosed, anticholinergic drugs for pain (although they may aggravate constipation), or faecal softeners to avoid obstructive episodes. Sublaxative doses of Senokot have been shown to be spasmolytic and might prove to have a place in management. Drugs to avoid are morphine, neostigmine, and the hypnotic glutethimide, which has been reported to cause smooth muscle spasm. Surgery may be needed in complicated cases.

Inflammatory disease of the large bowel

In the differential diagnosis of a patient with diarrhoea, abdominal pain, change in bowel habit, and rectal bleeding it is worth considering inflammatory conditions such as Crohn's disease and ulcerative coloproctitis. Though much rarer than carcinoma or diverticular disease, they are managed differently and have different treatment possibilities.

Crohn's disease and ulcerative coloproctitis

In the elderly Crohn's disease tends to affect the distal colon and rectum. It may present at first like diverticular disease, but persistent, modest bleeding from the rectum should suggest Crohn's disease rather than diverticulitis, in which rectal bleeding is more likely to be intermittent and severe. Local fistulas or extraintestinal complications suggest inflammatory disease rather than diverticular disease. Although the two conditions may coexist, Crohn's disease must be recognised when it is present. Management calls for steroid treatment; surgical intervention often leads to complications.

Ulcerative coloproctitis may appear for the first time in the elderly and is then often more persistent and has a worse prognosis than in younger subjects. Diagnosis is confirmed by endoscopy and biopsy, and management is along the usual lines, including steroid and sulphasalazine treatment.

Carcinoma of the large bowel

Carcinoma of the large bowel is mainly a disease of late middle and old age. Half of all cases occur in the distal colon, and over one third of these present with complete intestinal obstruction. A recent change in bowel habit is an important symptom; mucus or blood may also be passed per rectum. The value of routine rectal examination in elderly patients cannot be overemphasised. Bleeding is usually occult, and the patient may present with iron deficiency anaemia. This is common in old age, its most usual cause being gastrointestinal blood loss. Haemorrhoids may be secondary to a carcinoma higher up. Proctoscopy and sigmoidoscopy should precede a barium enema, which is unlikely to help unless clinical features – for example, bleeding, an abdominal mass, or sigmoidoscopic findings – point fairly clearly to the large gut.

Intestinal obstruction

Intestinal obstruction can be either mechanical or paralytic (adynamic). Mechanical obstructions are usually a surgical problem. They may lie in the small gut – for example, in hernia or adhesions – or in the large gut – for example, in carcinoma of the distal colon, diverticular disease, or volvulus of the colon. The major exception, not requiring surgery, is faecal impaction, which is easy to diagnose and amenable to medical treatment. Adynamic obstruction is seen in mesenteric vascular occlusion, ruptured aneurysm of the abdominal aorta, acute pancreatitis, and various other causes of peritonitis.

Gastrointestinal bleeding

Haematemesis and melaena may occur from a peptic ulcer, whether or not drugs, such as corticosteroids and non-steroidal anti-inflammatory drugs, have been taken. Haematemesis may also occur, though far less often, from hiatus hernia, reflux oesophagitis, oesophageal varices, the Mallory-Weiss syndrome, a gastric neoplasm, or a blood dyscrasia. Appreciable rectal bleeding is usually due to diverticular disease of the colon. Occult gastrointestinal bleeding may present as iron deficiency anaemia, and patients with iron deficiency anaemia should have serial consecutive faecal occult blood tests.

An association between calcific aortic stenosis and idiopathic lower gastrointestinal bleeding has been recognised for nearly 25 years and has recently been reviewed.[7] At the Mayo Clinic patients with this valvular lesion were around 100 times more likely to develop gastrointestinal bleeding than were the general clinic population.[8] In some cases arteriovenous malformations have been found in the right or left side of the colon or in the small bowel. If the patient is a suitable candidate for aortic valve replacement, this may be sufficient to cure the bleeding, but if aortic valve replacement is not indicated partial colectomy (usually right sided) may be needed.

Ischaemia of the intestine

There are three syndomes of intestinal ischaemia.

Acute mesenteric vascular occlusion – Acute mesenteric vascular occlusion (arterial or venous) produces the dramatic symptoms and signs associated with mesenteric infarction[9] – that is, acute abdominal pain, vomiting, and diarrhoea (perhaps bloodstained), distension with little guarding, loss of gut sounds, and shock. Pre-existing cardiac disease is common and may predispose to intestinal infarction without the presence of any obstruction of the mesenteric vessels. Nevertheless, arterial embolism or thrombosis are the most common lesions, the first usually being associated with atrial fibrillation. The prognosis is poor; massive resection of intestine gives poor results with a high mortality or nutritional problems if the patient survives. A direct attack on the artery is more hopeful, possibly aided by an arterial anastomotic procedure – for example, to the right common iliac artery.

Chronic intestinal ischaemia may produce either intestinal angina or ischaemic colitis. Intestinal angina presents characteristically with periumbilical pain soon after meals, unrelieved by alkalis[10]; the severity of the pain is related to the size of the meal so that meals get smaller and weight loss begins. Diarrhoea may also occur. A bruit may be heard in the epigastrium, but few other signs are found. Barium studies are negative, but aortography, with coeliac axis or superior mesenteric angiography, or both, will show the arterial lesions.

Ischaemic colitis results from more distal obstruction in mesenteric vessels, although both the small and large gut may be affected: the lesions are segmental. This diagnosis is worth while considering in the elderly with chronic diarrhoea without an obvious cause. Barium enema may help but, again, the diagnosis is best made by aortography. Some cases heal, though strictures may have developed. Conservative treatment is recommended if the diagnosis is certain (carcinoma having been excluded) unless complications, such as spreading peritonitis, ensue.[11] Ischaemic colitis has been reviewed by Saegesser *et al.*[12] Droller has reported 13 cases of atheromatous disease of the vessels supplying the gut in 1700 geriatric patients.[13]

Appendicitis

Though the clinical features of appendicitis are similar to those at younger ages, complications are found five times as often at operation: thus early diagnosis is vital.

Peptic ulceration

Peptic ulcer is common in the elderly. In women it is usually gastric, but in men the duodenal to gastric ratio of 4:1, which is seen at earlier ages, is maintained. It used to be taught that large gastric ulcers are probably malignant, but this can no longer be applied to the elderly, who may develop giant gastric ulcers that are benign and may heal rapidly. On the other hand, as the rate of recurrence is high and the risk of haemorrhage strong,[14] surgical intervention may still become necessary. Acute gastric erosions may be due to drugs, especially aspirin, which may be taken for conditions such as arthritis.

The history of peptic ulcer in the elderly is often atypical and may be short and without pain. A barium meal is often essential for making the diagnosis. If the results it yields suggest or at least do not exclude the possibility of malignancy fibreoscopy can also then be of value. An accurate diagnosis must be established because management (as always) depends on this. Biopsy or brush cytology may be obtained at endoscopy.

Treatment in the elderly should not include bed rest or strict dietary regimens because the first is unwise and the second usually impractical. Patients should avoid smoking, although some old people find this difficult. Alkalis and cholinergic drugs may be used with care. Carbenoxolone should be avoided because it tends to produce troublesome hypokalaemia in the elderly, especially those taking diuretics or with liver dysfunction. It may also give rise to salt and water retention, heart failure, and the need for further diuretic treatment. There have been no reports of fluid and electrolyte disturbances after the use of deglycyrrhizinised liquorice (Caved-S). De-Nol, a chelated bismuth compound, is said to protect the site of the ulcer and promote healing of both gastric and duodenal ulcers. Its use does not impose severe restrictions on diet, smoking, etc, and is reported not to disturb electrolyte balance. Maintenance treatment with De-Nol is not indicated, although an initial four week course may be repeated once if necessary.

In recent years H_2 receptor antagonists have been widely used to treat peptic ulcer, especially duodenal ulcer. These agents are suitable for long term maintenance treatment aimed at preventing the recurrence of peptic ulceration.

Cimetidine, introduced in 1976, crosses the blood-brain barrier and has produced neuropsychiatric adverse reactions in the elderly, especially those with impaired renal function or associated severe medical illness. Delirium or lesser degrees of confusion may occur, and reversible coma, hallucinations, paranoia, and depression have also been seen. Tranquillisers may add to the toxic confusional state. Pre-existing senile dementia of Alzheimer's type may be a predisposing factor, although symptoms that have been induced by drugs are probably then attributed to dementia. Intravenous physostigmine has reversed cimetidine-induced delerium.[15,16] Other side effects of cimetidine, which are well documented, include fever, leucopenia, rash, slurred speech, increased serum creatinine concentration, and antiandrogenic effects.[17] Cimetidine reduces hepatic blood flow and interacts with the hepatic cytochrome P450 in the drug metabolising enzyme system, thereby reducing the metabolism of certain other drugs – for example, diazepam, chlordiazepoxide, propranolol, theophylline, phenytoin, and warfarin – and increasing the risk of their toxicity. Cimetidine has an increased half life in the elderly, and the dose should be lower than for younger patients (for example, 300 mg twice daily). Ranitidine, a recent introduction, avoids many of the side effects attributed to cimetidine and therefore has advantages for the elderly patient.[18] Nevertheless, age related pharmacokinetic changes have been reported for ranitidine,[19] and interaction with theophylline has recently been described.[20]

Complications of peptic ulcer call for the usual prompt measures. Elderly patients are more likely to bleed from their peptic ulcers[21] and do not tolerate haemorrhage well, especially upper gastrointestinal bleeding.[22,23] Clinically, perforation may be remarkably silent in old people.[24]

Carcinoma of the stomach

The incidence of cancer of the stomach increases with age and is higher than the incidence that would be expected by chance when the cancer occurs in association with pernicious anaemia. Cancer of the stomach is often diagnosed late because of the insidious onset of anorexia and weight loss, and it should be suspected when investigating any anaemia. The results of faecal occult blood tests, barium meal, and, if indicated, fibre-endoscopy will help to form the diagnosis. Exfoliative cytology may be valuable, but studies of gastric acid are less so in the elderly, although the presence of free acid makes the diagnosis of cancer of the stomach less likely.

Disorders of the liver and gall bladder

Structural and functional changes in the liver and gall bladder occur with age.[25,26] Age related reduction in liver blood flow and certain enzyme functions have implications for drug treatment in the old.

Jaundice

The assessment and management of jaundice in elderly patients are essentially the same as in younger patients. Gall stones, side effect of drugs, and obstruction by neoplasm are the diagnoses usually suspected in elderly patients with jaundice. Nevertheless, a fact worth remembering is that the most common cause of jaundice in the elderly with congestive cardiac failure is pulmonary infarction. This occurs because the increased pigment derived from the liberated haemoglobin in the infarct overloads the anoxic liver cells.

Obstructive jaundice is more common than hepatocellular jaundice, and extrahepatic obstruction (due to neoplasm or gall stones) is more common than intrahepatic obstruction (caused by cholestasis, which is usually drug induced). The most common cause of obstructive jaundice is neoplasm, which is usually carcinoma of the head of the pancreas but sometimes metastatic neoplastic deposits in the liver or in the lymph nodes at the porta hepatis. Primary carcinomas of the gall bladder and bile ducts or of the liver itself are rare.

Calculous obstruction of the common bile duct may be a painless illness in the elderly. As pain and even a fluctuating depth of jaundice may occur in malignant cases, differential diagnosis can be difficult. Effort should be made to avoid undue delay in establishing the diagnosis as the mortality may then rise sharply. If the diagnosis has not been established within six weeks after the onset of jaundice in an elderly patient laparotomy should be performed. Modern techniques of liver imaging will often help to avoid delays of this length in diagnosis.[26]

Hepatitis and cirrhosis

Hepatitis in older patients is not common but has a graver prognosis than in younger patients. It can be difficult to diagnose and may even lead to unnecessary laparotomy if it causes obstructive jaundice. Serum hepatitis is insidious in onset and affects patients who are older and iller than those affected by infectious hepatitis, although this tends to assume a more virulent character in the old than in the young.

Cirrhosis is not rare but may be clinically latent and is usually cryptogenic in old age. Primary biliary cirrhosis is sometimes seen in elderly women, who present with pruritus and, later, jaundice, malabsorption, pigmentation, xanthomata, clubbing, and hepato-splenomegaly. Haemochromatosis is occasionally seen in the elderly and may be associated with polyarthritis.

Drugs

Drugs may adversely affect the liver, causing hepatic necrosis, fatty liver, a hepatitis like reaction, or intrahepatic cholestasis (sometimes due to hypersensitivity).

The table sets out various causes and categories of liver injury and gives examples relevant to elderly patients. In geriatric practice the main drugs implicated are: phenothiazines (especially chlor-promazine), antidepressants, oral hypoglycaemic agents, anti-rheumatic drugs, antituberculous drugs, sulphonamides, diuretics, antithyroid drugs, anticonvulsants, dichloralphenazone, and oral anabolic agents. Elderly patients who need anabolic agents should be given them by intramuscular injection – for example, Deca-Durabolin every three weeks – rather than by mouth.

Gall stones

The incidence of gall stones increases with age, especially in women. Symptoms are due to complications, which develop more often in the elderly, who then fare less well than younger patients. Apart from diagnostic difficulties, surgery under non-elective conditions carries a relatively high mortality. The most common problem faced is probably that of silent gall stones, in which, despite the risk of complications, most authors advocate a con-servative approach in patients over 60. Some patients may be suitable for dissolution of gall stones by oral treatment – for example, administration of chenodeoxycholic or ursodeoxycholic acid.[27,28]

Cholecystitis

Cholecystitis is usually associated with gall stones. Acute attacks may mimic other abdominal emergencies, myocardial infarction, or pleurisy. Treatment is by antibiotics with supportive treatments. Rifamide, an antibiotic that is concentrated in bile, may be useful; otherwise a bactericidal broad spectrum antibiotic, such as ampicillin

Examples of toxic liver injury in elderly patients

Mechanism of injury	Toxic agents	
	Drugs	Other agents
Hepatic necrosis	Halogenated hydro-carbons	Dicophane (DDT)
	Heavy metals	Paraquat
	Cytotoxic drugs	Benzene derivatives
	Intravenous tetra-cycline	Amanita mushrooms
	Overdose of iron or paracetamol	Irradiation
		Burns
		Hyperpyrexia
Fatty liver	Alcohol	Various organic and inorganic chemicals
		Irradiation
		Other diseases, such as ulcerative colitis, diabetes, anaemia
Hepatitis like reaction	Antidepressants	
	Anticonvulsants	
	Antituberculous drugs	
	Antirheumatic drugs	
	Halothane	
Intrahepatic cholestasis due to hypersensitivity	Chlorpromazine	
	Antidepressants	
	Oral hypoglycaemic agents	
	Benzodiazepines	
	Thiazides	
	Phenylbutazone	
	Antithyroid drugs	
	Sulphonamides	
Intrahepatic cholestasis without hypersensitivity	Methyltestosterone	
	Oral anabolic agents	
Mixed	Antituberculous drugs	
	Sulphonamides	
	Oral antidiabetic agents	
	Methyldopa	
	Erythromycin estolate	

or cephaloridine, should be used. Erythromycin estolate should be avoided, as should morphine. Complications, which include gangrene, perforation, or empyema of the gall bladder, are more likely in the elderly. British surgeons tend to be cautious about cholecystectomy soon after acute cholecystitis, but American and Scandinavian surgeons favour intervention early after the acute stage. The wisdom of early surgery in the elderly has, however, been questioned.[29]

Chronic cholecystitis associated with gall stones, which it usually is, is the most common disease of the biliary system. The onset is usually insidious, and symptoms, which are vague, include: "flatulent dyspepsia," especially after fatty food; nausea and vomiting; and discomfort in the right hypochondrium (or right scapula or shoulder). There may be tenderness over the gall bladder and a positive Murphy's sign. The picture is often atypical and must be distinguished from hiatus hernia and peptic ulcer, colonic disorders, and urinary infections. Oral cholecystography can be remarkably unhelpful in the elderly. Treatment may be medical, using weight reduction and restriction of fat intake, but it is then symptomatic; the definitive treatment if stones are present is cholecystectomy.

[1] Standeven A. The acute abdomen in the elderly. *Practitioner* 1979; **222**: 465–70.
[2] Clark ANG. Deficiency states in duodenal diverticular disease. *Age Ageing* 1972; **1**; 14–23.
[3] Parks, TG. Natural history of diverticular disease in the colon. *Clin Gastroenterol* 1975; **4**: 53–69.
[4] Painter NS, Burkitt DP. Diverticular disease of the colon: deficiency disease of Western civilisation. *Br Med J* 1971; ii: 450–4.
[5] Parks TG, Connell AM, Gough AD, *et al.* Limitations of radiology in the differentiation of diverticulitis and diverticulosis of the colon. *Br Med J* 1970; ii: 136–8.
[6] Painter NS. Diverticular disease. *Br Med J* 1971; ii: 156.
[7] Shbeeb I, Prager E, Love J. The aortic valve: colonic axis. *Dis Colon Rectum* 1984; **27**: 38–41.
[8] Cody MC, O'Donovan TP, Hughes RW Jr. Idiopathic gastrointestinal bleeding and aortic stenosis. *Am J Dig Dis* 1974; **19**: 393–8.
[9] Jackson BB. *Occlusion of the superior mesenteric artery.* Springfield Illinois: CC Thomas, 1963.
[10] Dick AP, Graff R, Gregg DM, *et al.* An arteriographic study of mesenteric arterial disease. *Gut* 1967; **8**: 206–20.
[11] Marcuson RW, Farman JA. Ischaemic disease of the colon. *Proc R Soc Med* 1971; **64**: 1080–3.
[12] Saegesser F, Roenspies U, Robinson JW. Ischaemic diseases of the large intestine. *Pathobiol Ann* 1979; **9**: 303–37.
[13] Droller H. Atheromatous disease of the vessels supplying the gut. *Age Ageing* 1972; **1**: 162–7.
[14] Strange SL. Giant innocent gastric ulcer in the elderly. *Gerontologia Clinica* 1963; **5**: 171–89.
[15] Mogelnicki SR, Waller JL, Finlayson DC. Physostigmine reversal of cimetidine-induced mental confusion. *JAMA* 1979; **241**: 826–7.
[16] Jenike MA. Cimetidine in elderly patients: review of uses and risks. *J Am Geriatr Soc* 1982; **30**: 170–3.
[17] Cimetidine (Tagamet): update on adverse effects. *Med Let Drugs Ther* 1978; **20**: 77–80.
[18] Richards DA. Comparative pharmacodynamics and pharma cokinetics of cimetidine and ranitidine. *J Clin Gastroenterol* 1983; **5**, suppl 1: 81–90.

[19] Hockings NF, Stevenson IH. The effect of age and renal function on ranitidine disposition. *Journal of Clinical and Experimental Gerontology* 1982; **4**: 267–75.

[20] Fernandes E, Melewicz FM. Ranitidine and theophylline. *Ann Intern Med* 1984; **100**: 459.

[21] Allan R, Dykes P. A study of the factors influencing mortality rates from gastrointestinal haemorrhage. *Q J Med* 1976; **45**: 533–50.

[22] Jones FA. Hematemesis and melena with special reference to causation and to factors influencing mortality from bleeding peptic ulcers. *Gastroenterology* 1956; **30**: 166–90.

[23] Altman DF. Gastrointestinal diseases in the elderly. *Med Clin North Am* 1983; **67**: 433–44.

[24] Coleman JA, Denham MJ. Perforation of peptic ulceration in the elderly. *Age Ageing* 1980; **9**: 257–61.

[25] Earnest DL, MacGregor IL. Therapy for gastrointestinal disease. In: Conrad K, Bressler R, eds. *Drug therapy for the elderly*. St Louis: CV Mosby, 1981: 159–209.

[26] Hyams DE. The liver and biliary system. In: Platt D, ed. *Geriatrics 2*. Berlin: Springer-Verlag, 1983: 45–85.

[27] Bouchier IAD. Gall stone dissolving agents. *Br Med J* 1983; **286**: 778–80.

[28] Dowling RH. Cholelithiasis: medical treatment. *Clin Gastroenterol* 1983; **12**: 125–78.

[29] Norrby S, Heuman R, Sjödahl R. Early and late results after early cholecystectomy in acute cholecystitis with special reference to the age factor. *Journal of Clinical and Experimental Gerontology* 1983; **5**: 323–36.

Rehabilitation of the elderly

H M HODKINSON

Rehabilitation of the elderly patient – that is, helping him to resume as normal a life as possible (preferably in his own home) – is a vital part of his treatment. Particular problems are raised if the elderly patient has to be admitted to hospital because the traditional patterns of care are poorly suited to the needs of the elderly, which can create problems when it comes to rehabilitation. Nursing in bed is central to the traditional pattern of care; however, the dangers of going to bed, which have been brilliantly expounded by Richard Asher,[1] apply with particular force to the elderly. Other problems are raised by the dangerous institutionalising effects of staying in hospital, where the "good" patient is the one who readily allows himself to be regimented and accepts the role of a passive yet grateful recipient of care. The important goals of self care are removed: clothes are replaced by dressing gown and slippers, so emphasising the patient's role as the invalid; and the patient is further conditioned to dependency by a plethora of professionals, whose authoritarian status is enhanced by such devices as hierarchies and uniforms. The end result is the patient who, when management decisions are put to him, says, "You know best, doctor, I leave it all to you" and unquestioningly accepts being treated rather like a slow witted child, allowing things to be done for him that he could perfectly well do for himself. Here again, the elderly are perhaps more vulnerable to these institutionalising pressures, being undervalued members of the community and survivors from a more authoritarian age.

Underexpectation presents another problem. Elderly patients and their relatives, friends, and neighbours and, regrettably, sometimes their general practitioners too tend to have an unduly pessimistic view of the likely outcome of the admission to hospital. Their outdated view of the hospital, not rarely a former workhouse with perhaps a previously unenviable local reputation, is that an old person came out of it only one way – feet first. Thus we

54

constantly hear such remarks as, "What can you expect at my age, doctor?" from elderly patients. These prejudices need to be forcefully counteracted as the benefits of hospital treatment for old people can stand comparison with those for younger age groups,[2] and most elderly patients can be discharged home again after treatment in an active geriatric department.[3-5] Day hospitals can avoid some of the disadvantages of inpatient care, and rehabilitation is a major component of their work.[6]

Creating the right atmosphere

Successful rehabilitation needs an appropriate atmosphere of activity and optimism. This depends on many different groups: other patients; relatives; nurses; doctors; voluntary helpers; ward orderlies; porters; ministers of religion; social workers; and paramedical therapists. This large group of individuals forms a "therapeutic community," and this, and not just the rehabilitation team of physiotherapists, occupational therapists, speech therapists, and doctors, determines the quality of rehabilitation. Good communication is needed if rehabilitation is to thrive. The nursing sister, paramedical therapists, and medical staff have important roles as group leaders and need to create and maintain the right attitudes of enthusiasm and optimism around them; help and direct others in the application of rehabilitative techniques; and give support and encouragement to all the members of the therapeutic community.

Creating the appropriate atmosphere for rehabilitation in a hospital ward is greatly facilitated by its specialised geriatric function, which is possibly the chief justification for the separation of geriatrics from general medicine. Seeing other patients improve and go home is without doubt an encouragement to the individual patient. Thus the more active departments have an advantage in this respect,[3-5] but systems of progressive patient care are practised in most departments whereby long stay patients are transferred to other accommodation in order to maintain greater activity in the admission and rehabilitation wards.

Role of nursing staff

Nursing staff play a vital part in rehabilitation. Because of their close contact with patients, relatives, and visitors they can best communicate that the department has a therapeutic as opposed to a custodial orientation. Nursing attitudes and practice must be adapted to the elderly. Rather than simply ministering to the patient, the geriatric nurse needs to help him to help himself and so foster increasing independence. Firm but sympathetic re-education may be needed to modify the patient's expectations. Overprotective attitudes must be abandoned; "Don't you walk on your own, you might fall" may negate all that the physiotherapist has done to build up skill and confidence in walking. Nurses should be intimately involved in the rehabilitation of the patient so that they know what stage the physiotherapist or occupational therapist has reached and can supplement what is being done. Otherwise, wily old patients often have the nurse lifting and supporting them when they are quite capable of getting up unaided and walking with only supervision by the physiotherapist; or the nurse may be undressing and helping them into bed when earlier in the occupational therapy department they had dressed themselves and got in and out of bed unaided.

The elderly patient in need of rehabilitation may have a specific disability, such as hemiplegia, parkinsonism, or arthritis, but usually, rather than having a major specific disability, the patient needs to be able to resume normal activities after a period of illness, particularly when this has entailed bed rest, which has resulted in impairment of balance, walking, and other basic skills.

In assessing the individual patient's potential for improvement full and accurate evaluation of his physical disabilities is clearly important, but it must be coupled with full consideration of mental factors and the social background. Mental factors are of paramount importance, for well motivated patients with intact intelligence can often overcome the most daunting physical disabilities while patients with poor motivation, depression, or dementia may do badly, even with fairly minor physical disabilities. Routine assessment of intellectual function by a simple orientation and memory questionnaire may be valuable in planning the patient's rehabilitation.[7] Social factors determine what the specific aims of treatment should be – for example, whether the patient needs to be able to climb stairs or cook for himself – and what degree of self care is essential. Social factors may have a bearing on motivation, and returning home is the goal of most patients. Some may have to accept more restricted goals, such as admission to a welfare home, and the social worker may need to help patients to adjust to such changes without losing heart. We may have to accept, however, that the patient wants to go back to a home that is far from ideal; we may destroy his motivation if we persuade him too strenuously to accept some alternative plan that seems more satisfactory to us.

Basic requirements

Each patient will require something different from his programme of rehabilitation. Nevertheless, most will want to acquire the ability to walk with or without mechanical aids; to get up and down from a chair and in and out of bed; to manage the lavatory; and to dress. The patient may also need to use the stairs, cook, and do other household tasks. The occupational therapist is concerned with determining these needs, which are known as the activities of daily living (ADL), and in retraining the patient to the necessary standards. If necessary, the occupational therapist may arrange modifications to the home, changes in clothing (zips or Velcro to replace difficult buttons, for example), or the provision of gadgets to simplify difficult tasks (for example, a wide variety of gadgets to enable patients with hemiplegia to do tasks with one hand instead of two). Severely disabled patients may need extensive re-education and training, but more often patients can regain their confidence simply by going through and briefly practising their activities of daily living.

Remobilisation is the principal concern of the physiotherapist. If treatment does not start as soon as possible strength, confidence, morale, and balance may all deteriorate rapidly – for example, rehabilitation of patients with stroke starts as soon as consciousness has returned. The patient practises rising from a chair, with a seat of suitable height, by pushing strongly on its arms while leaning well forwards with feet kept under the front edge of the chair. If needed, help is given by lifting with the hand under the axilla. The walking frame is commonly used when practising walking as it gives patients considerable support and confidence. The following simple gait pattern may be taught: the frame is advanced about 18 in (45 cm) and planted securely; the patient takes a short step with each foot; stops; and advances the frame to repeat the cycle. Even this simple regimen may call for repeated instruction of confused patients; indeed, the essential principles of geriatric rehabilitation are simplicity, consistency, and repetition. Initially a helper at each side may be needed, but patients generally make rapid progress to walking in the frame independently. This level of activity may be the most that can be expected from very disabled patients, but for other patients progress to a stick and ultimately no aid is typically smooth, and patients do not become "addicted" to their frame if their rehabilitation is satisfactorily directed. In hemiplegics who can grip with only one hand the less satisfactory tripod may have to be used rather than a frame.

In geriatric rehabilitation stimulation of the patient's motivation and showing approval of success are important, and the therapist's main tool is her own personality, not complicated apparatus or techniques. Some patients, particularly during the early stages of their rehabilitation, need to be put under considerable pressure by the therapist to augment their poor motivation. The successful therapist is the one who can support, encourage, and if necessary push the patient hard without alienating him, and flexibly adapt her approach to the personality of the patient.

Maintaining improvement at home

When the elderly patient leaves hospital or day hospital the level of activity achieved by rehabilitation needs to be maintained. Follow up at home – for example, by the health visitor or geriatric nurse visitor, can help to ensure that overprotective relatives or friends do not encourage a retreat into dependency. Attendance at a day centre or other social activities can provide incentive and stimulus.

Modifications of the home may be helpful – for example, fixing handrails or providing more suitable toilet facilities – or more suitable chairs, wheelchairs, or bath aids may be necessary. Local authorities employ domiciliary occupational therapists to help in such matters. Moving the bed downstairs may be a great help, but this should not be done without careful thought because many old people who walk poorly on the level manage stairs well because of the help from the stair rails. Bringing down the bed may encourage the invalid role and at the same time cause unnecessary major inconvenience to other members of the family.

Though this account of rehabilitation of the elderly has concentrated on the part played by hospital treatment, the general practitioner also has an important part to play. He can be the most powerful influence in the re-education of the elderly and their relatives so that they become less pessimistic and more aware of the potential benefits of inpatient rehabilitation. This will be best accomplished if the general practitioner is supported by an active geriatric service with no waiting list. He can then help his elderly patients by making early referrals rather than waiting until a crisis has developed; instead of accepting that advancing disability is just an inevitable concomitant of aging he can regard it as a diagnostic and therapeutic challenge.

[1] Asher R. *Richard Asher talking sense.* Jones FA, ed. London: Pitman Medical, 1972.
[2] Arnold J, Exton-Smith AN. The geriatric department and the community. Value of hospital treatment in the elderly. *Lancet* 1962; ii: 551–3.
[3] Hodkinson HM, Jefferys PM. Making hospital geriatrics work. *Br Med J* 1972; iv: 536–9.

4 O'Brien TD, Joshi DM, Warren EW. No apology for geriatrics. *Br Med J* 1973; iv: 277–80.

5 Bagnall WE, Datta SR, Knox J, Horrocks P. Geriatric medicine in Hull: a comprehensive service. *Br Med J* 1977; ii: 102–4.

6 Brocklehurst JC, Tucker JS. Progress in geriatric day care. London: King Edward's Hospital Fund for London, 1980.

7 Hodkinson HM. Evaluation of a mental test score for assessment of mental impairment in the elderly. *Age Ageing* 1972; 1: 233–8.

Non-specific presentation of illness in the elderly

H M HODKINSON

Presentation of illness in the elderly often differs misleadingly from that in younger age groups, particularly as it can be entirely non-specific. Some differences in the elderly may reflect altered responses in certain mechanisms – for instance, those responsible for producing fever or pain. For example, myocardial infarction may occur in the elderly without typical transverse chest pain and shock. Often pain is totally absent, and the patient presents with an episode of collapse, confusion, or breathlessness. Similarly, lobar pneumonia in the young is indicated by cough, fever, and leucocytosis but in the elderly it may present insidiously with confusion, drowsiness, unsteadiness, and slight breathlessness. These vague patterns of illness are often seen in the elderly; this chapter will consider some of the more common presenting syndromes.

"Failure to thrive"

Illness often presents as an insidious and progressive physical deterioration, which is aptly described by the paediatric term "failure to thrive." Typically, the patient's decline comprises deteriorating social competence, loss of appetite and weight, increasing frailty, and diminishing initiative, concentration, and drive. This general failure of the old person is all too often accepted as being due to old age or senility or is regarded as a dementing process, while the physical basis is overlooked. There are many diagnostic possibilities.

Malignant disease

Malignant disease in the elderly quite often presents in this way – that is, as a failure to thrive. The common primary sites are the lung, breast, prostate, colon, and rectum. A chest x ray film and rectal examination, with examination of the breasts in women, are therefore essential parts of the assessment of the elderly patient with an unexplained general deterioration. Diagnosis may lead to useful treatment: endocrine treatment is often helpful in cancer of the breast or prostate, even when metastasis is present, while resection may be of benefit in colorectal growths.

Endocrine and metabolic disorders

Endocrine and metabolic disorders should also be considered. Thyroid disease is particularly difficult to recognise clinically in the old. In a series of geriatric patients with hypothyroidism only 28 % showed the classic picture of myxoedema while 54 % had a totally non-specific presentation.[1] Similarly, hyperthyroidism is often atypical in its clinical presentation.[2] It may present with physical lethargy and mental depression or with general debility, perhaps accompanied by cardiac failure and sometimes auricular fibrillation, but with none of the other usual stigmata of thyrotoxicosis. The fairly high prevalence, difficulty of clinical recognition, and treatable nature of thyroid disease makes a strong case for performing thyroid function tests routinely in ill old people.

Diabetes is another common disease that may also produce failure to thrive rather than present classically. It is easily missed as glycosuria may not occur owing to high renal threshold; thus a random blood sugar measurement provides a much more reliable screening test.[3] Uraemia, which is a further diagnostic possibility, is most often due to chronic pyelonephritis.

Thus in old people who fail to thrive performing laboratory screening tests is of great value. Among the most useful would be measurements of blood urea, electrolyte, glucose, and haemoglobin concentrations and thyroid function tests.

Diseases of the central nervous system

Diseases of the central nervous system may also present unobtrusively. Although parkinsonism occurs commonly in old age, it is often missed because tremor is either absent or slight and the typical rigidity may not be noticed. Doctors should actively look for the disease because treatment with L-dopa can often make a worthwhile contribution. Multiple minor strokes and the development of a pseudobulbar syndrome are less likely to be overlooked. Ignoring peripheral neuropathy is occasionally a pitfall as malignant disease or diabetes is the most common cause of this condition.

Depression

Depression is another possible cause of failure to thrive that is often overlooked both in general practice and in hospital. Depression is common in old age but may often present an atypical picture, masquerading as physical disease or as failure to thrive. The possibility of depression must always be kept in mind by doctors dealing with the elderly. Inquiring about the cardinal symptoms of depression – namely, early waking and anorexia – may often show this to be the diagnosis, while further questioning of the apparently cheerful old person may uncover gross depression or suicidal ideas. Depression in the old is usually treated with one of the tricyclic or quadricyclic antidepressants, and the results are often gratifying.

Chronic infections

Chronic infections are a more unusual cause of insidious decline. Nevertheless, though uncommon, pulmonary tuberculosis (particularly in elderly men) and subacute bacterial endocarditis should be remembered as possible causes because they are serious but also potentially treatable.

Iatrogenic illness

Iatrogenic illness should always be considered because the elderly are particularly vulnerable to the adverse effects of drugs.[3] The side effects of drugs that can present as failure to thrive include: hangover from over sedation with hypnotics (particularly those with longer half lives); drug induced depression; drug induced parkinsonism from phenothiazines; and severe hyponatraemia from carbamazepine, chlorpropamide, or long term use of thiazide diuretics.

Falls and blackouts

Falls and blackouts are important presenting features in the elderly that often lead to hospital admission because of resultant trauma or fracture. Patients with parkinsonism are particularly prone to repeated falls, and so are those with unstable knees from osteoarthritis. Patients with rheumatoid arthritis affecting the cervical spine may have falls because of the vertebrobasilar insufficiency that occurs on moving the neck. So called "premonitory falls" may herald acute physical illness such as pneumonia.

The side effects of drugs must also be included on the list of causes. Hypotensive drugs are commonly to blame for falls and blackouts and all too often these have been prescribed on flimsy grounds, the patient not having true sustained hypertension. The mechanism is that of postural hypotension, which may also result from overenthusiastic treatment with diuretics that has lowered the serum sodium concentration. Oversedation with hypnotics or tranquillisers may also result in falls.

Mental deterioration

Physical illness presents very often as mental disturbance in the elderly patient, and such mental symptoms must not be mistakenly ascribed to dementia or "senility." The possibility of a physical cause will obviously be considered most carefully when the mental symptoms are of recent onset.

Acute confusional states

Acute confusional states may be due to a wide variety of diseases,[4] but the most important are lobar pneumonia, bronchopneumonia, urinary infection, cardiac failure, and left ventricular failure. Though confusional states may readily occur in patients whose previous mental state was completely normal, pre-existing dementia and parkinsonism both appear to facilitate their development.[4] Drug treatment may also result in confusional states: hypnotics, antidepressants, and anti-parkinsonian drugs are especially noteworthy. Among the anti-parkinsonian drugs the older atropine like drugs, such as benzhexol and orphenadrine, are troublesome, but amantadine can produce confusional states that are remarkable for their intense visual hallucinations. Subacute and chronic confusional states are particularly likely to be mistaken for dementia, and here causes such as uraemia, carcinomatosis, pernicious anaemia, or hypothyroidism should be considered.

Organic brain disease may result in true dementia. In some instances an accurate diagnosis – for example, that of cerebral arteriosclerosis or cerebral tumour – may not lead to any possible treatments, but the diagnosis of rarer diseases, such as subdural haematoma, low pressure hydrocephalus, or general paresis can be important because they are potentially reversible.

"Rheumatism"

Because of the high incidence of degenerative joint disease poorly localised skeletal or muscular aches and pains are so common in old age that "rheumatic" pains heralding treatable or serious disease may unwisely be ignored. Osteomalacia is an important example: it is far from rare, eminently treatable, but easily overlooked. It particularly affects the housebound, those with previous gastric surgery, and women rather than men. The patient becomes progressively more disabled, with "rheumatic" pains and proximal muscle weakness as the key symptoms. They may develop a typical gait (like a waddling "penguin") and find getting up from a chair particularly difficult because of muscle weakness.

Another important cause of "rheumatic" pain is the presence of metastases in bone. These occur most commonly from carcinoma of the breast or prostate and for a time may respond well to hormonal treatment. Deposits of multiple myeloma are another possible cause of the pain. Recently developed severe low back pain in an elderly person is quite commonly caused by these conditions whereas it is rarely accounted for by prolapse of the intervertebral disc or a simple osteoporotic collapse.

Immobility

An old person "going off his feet" is a common reason for admission to a geriatric department. Again, all too often this is simply blamed on old age and the physical basis is overlooked. Disease of the central nervous system, especially strokes or parkinsonism, and locomotor disease, such as osteoarthritis, rheumatoid arthritis, or osteomalacia, are major causes of immobility. Fracture is quite often overlooked as the cause for immobility in patients who have had many falls. Immobility may also develop because of general frailty in the context of failure to thrive or because of loss of confidence due to repeated falls or unsteadiness – for example, from laterally unstable knees in severe osteoarthritis, postural hypotension, or oversedation.

Incontinence

Incontinence too should not automatically be accepted as due to old age or mental deterioration. Immobility itself may cause incontinence, and other major factors are: urinary infection; urinary retention with overflow; stress incontinence in old women who have had children; faecal impaction giving rise to either urinary retention or spurious diarrhoea and faecal incontinence; and incontinence associated with the urgency caused by diuretic treatment. Night sedation may be responsible for incontinence during the night.

Conclusion

All these examples show that presentation is often misleading or obscure in elderly patients, a factor which calls for special vigilance. Unless full use is made of good history taking (particularly with regard to drug treatment), physical examination, and relevant investigations, many errors will be made. The non-specific presentation of illness in the old must be regarded as a diagnostic challenge. If this attitude is adopted medical work with the elderly becomes a fascinating, exacting, and rewarding discipline. Only by proper diagnosis can the elderly be helped to the full. If their symptoms are dismissed as "old age," "senility," "rheumatism," or if some other conveniently vague label is applied many opportunities for effective treatment of old patients will be missed at the cost of much unnecessary suffering and disability.

[1] Bahemuka M, Hodkinson HM. Screening for hypothyroidism in elderly in-patients. *Br Med J* 1975; ii: 601–3.

[2] Rønnov-Jessen V, Kirkegaard C. Hypothyroidism, a disease of old age? *Br Med J* 1973; i: 41–3.

[3] Royal College of Physicians. Medication for the elderly. *J R Coll Physicians Lond* 1984; **18**: 3–10.

[4] Hodkinson HM. Mental impairment in the elderly. *J R Coll Physicians Lond* 1973; 7: 307–17.

Care of the elderly in general practice

CHARLES HODES

Elderly people account for just over 15% of the population, and projections predict a similar proportion of elderly people in the year 2000, but within that proportion the older age groups, especially those over 85, are expected to increase. In 1981 a general practitioner with a list size of 2500 would have had approximately 233 patients aged 65–74, 120 aged 75–84, and 27 aged 84 and over. By the turn of the century a general practitioner with a similar list size could expect to have 193 patients in the 65 to 74 age group, 123 between 75 and 84, and 38 over the age of 85.[1] The development of the health team in recent years has enabled the general practitioner to approach the care of the elderly more from the point of view of prevention and early diagnosis,[2–4] and new developments with social workers and community psychiatric nurses in general practice[5] are bringing further benefits.

The assessment of the patient's needs and the organisation of the care required are the essential tasks of the general practitioner. These needs may be known or unknown to the patient. At least six different aspects should be considered.

The primary care team

The general practitioner, the health visitor, and the district nurse together can provide the best care for the elderly in their own home. Working from a common centre and sharing one medical record, there is adequate opportunity for exchange of information, which is so important in giving personal medical care to patients who often have some degree of mental confusion in addition to the usual spectrum of diseases. Age is not a barrier to attendance at the surgery, and in fact the elderly patient should be encouraged to remain mobile and attend as required. Consultation with the health visitor and treatment by the district nurse should also be available at the surgery. Appointments – making and keeping – are easily overlooked by the elderly, and it helps if they are always given an appointment in writing and a sympathetic receptionist fits them in without too much waiting if an appointment has not been made. Though willing relatives and friends may help increasingly with their own cars, more organised transport services in general practice are required if the preventive approach is to increase.

Information about the services available locally should be kept at every practice. Local authorities often have booklets of services and can provide well illustrated pamphlets on such subjects as diet and exercise; the health visitor is of course the best person to give out this information and can supplement it with individual consultation and with patient groups. Group discussions are also helpful in preparing for retirement[6]; health education for the elderly should include advice on prevention of accidents and fire safety. Local clubs, laundry services, washing facilities, chiropody, and meals on wheels are generally available and should be introduced to patients even if required only occasionally. Convalescent holidays are especially worth while for the elderly and whenever possible should cater for both husband and wife.

The nurse's role

The nurse has been identified increasingly with the care of the elderly sick patient, and 9% of the elderly received visits from the district nurse in 1979.[7] She can be supported in her work in the home by bath attendants and male nurses, who are playing an increasingly important part in the care of the male geriatric patient. Night nursing may also be available and, if required only short term, can make hospital admission unnecessary. Visits to the home for routine injections may also be important as a method of surveillance, and changes can be reported to other members of the team.

At present there is little in the way of domiciliary physiotherapy, but the district nurse can give help with breathing exercises for chest infection and continuing support for the patient with a hemiplegia. Aids to nursing, such as commodes, bed rests, and disposable bedding supplies, are always available. Laboratory services are now used extensively by general practitioners, and the district nurse can take urine and blood specimens in the home and return them to the surgery for collection by the hospital transport services. For haemoglobin estimation a Spence haemoglobinometer is very simple and quick to use, in both the home and surgery, and when any anaemia is due to poor diet the health visitor can soon call at home with advice and help.

Practice premises

Practice premises have changed considerably in recent years, and very large centres may present problems for the older patient. Cars should be able to drive up to the front entrance of the building, the doors should be wide enough for a wheelchair, and preferably there should be no steps. When all the members of the team have their own accommodation in the building referral is simpler and joint consultation can deal with problems quickly. A sufficient number of warm examination rooms allow the patients to dress and undress at their usual speed, and they can be helped by a receptionist or nurse; this also permits the general practitioner to carry on with other duties.

Good communication is facilitated by regular meetings between members of the primary care team. A high standard of record keeping is important, and the problem orientated record[8] may be found useful in geriatric care. All patients should keep with them at all times a treatment card that can be used for repeat prescriptions and give useful information to any doctor seeing the patient as an emergency without the medical record being available.

Studies on the unreported needs of old people[9] and an evaluation of early diagnostic services for the elderly[10] have indicated the need for preventive care. To carry this out in general practice requires an age-sex register from which the geriatric register can be constructed.[11,12] Invitations for examinations can be sent to selected patients, and these screening examinations can be carried out by the primary care team in the surgery and in the home; treatment and follow up are carried out as required. Special registers for high risk groups, such as patients living alone and the surviving partner on the death of a spouse, are indicated.

Social services

The elderly patient depends on the social services as well as the primary medical care team to live in the community. The social worker's client and the general practitioner's patient are the same person, and working together can only improve the total care of the elderly. If the social worker can use the general practitioner's premises regular communication is more likely and the preventive approach possible. The many benefits now available in the way of financial help and housing are best dealt with by the social worker. Psychogeriatric cases need the support of the social work services, and patients recently discharged from hospital can be followed by a worker who is in close contact with the psychiatric services. The home help, in addition to cleaning and shopping duties, is a great support for the often depressed and isolated patient and can alert the general practitioner if there is any deterioration. Selected personal social services to those over 65 include 8% having home helps, 2% meals on wheels, 3% lunch (lunch club or day centre), and 4% attending a day centre.[13]

When the elderly patient can no longer manage at home the social worker will arrange alternative accommodation. This may be in a flat or bungalow with a supervising warden. If this is not sufficient residential accommodation can be provided on a temporary or permanent basis. The temporary care may be used when a relative has to go into hospital or goes off on holiday; it may also be used for day care when meals are provided and occupational therapy is available. This also relieves the isolation of the permanent residents, bringing them into contact with their community, and introduces the temporary residents to what might become their home.

By arrangement with the local authority the general practitioner may provide medical care for the residents. In this work he can be supported by the health visitor and district nurse. It is useful to have an assessment chart for patients, in addition to the usual medical records, that can be shared by the primary medical care team. The chart is used to record essential information about the patients and to note changes that occur with time. The first part can be completed by the health visitor and gives a score based on assessments of physical state, mental state, activity, mobility, and incontinence. If the score rises the patient is deteriorating. The second part is completed by the nurse on admission and then periodically as indicated; there is a scoring system for hearing and the state of the feet.

Medical services

The geriatrician and his social worker in the local hospital are now very much part of community care and should be well known by the general practitioner. Domiciliary visits should be readily available without undue delay and requested for assessment and opinion, not only for admission. This prevents crises from developing and allows the geriatrician to plan his admissions. The increase in the numbers of psychogeriatric patients in general practice gives rise to problems of regular medication and also to overdosage; close supervision is required of patients living alone. The inclusion of geriatric and psychiatric services in district hospitals will strengthen the support given to general practitioners.

Refractive errors are common, and old spectacles may have been worn for many years; simple tests for visual acuity can be done in general practice, but the detection of glaucoma requires special equipment and should be carried out by an ophthalmologist. During school holidays a technician with suitable equipment may be "borrowed" from the local authority for sight testing in old people's homes. Hearing aids are usually given out by special centres and often require further travel for examination and fitting; patients of any age may benefit from an aid, and there should be regular supervision of its use and performance.

The community

The elderly patient usually wishes to continue to be independent and is supported by family and neighbours. The general practitioner can help by providing and introducing skilled help. The voluntary societies such as the British Red Cross and Women's Royal Voluntary Service and help given by local groups such as Rotary clubs are most valuable. Group practices and health centres can have groups of "friends," who give help of all kinds to the elderly.

The patient

Old people often do not come forward for care – medical or social. This reluctance may be less in relation to the family doctor who is a familiar face, and the health visitor and nurse working with him are identified by the patient as part of the same care. Altogether 66.2% of the over 75s consulted their general practitioners during the course of a year.[14] An understanding of the patient's attitude is therefore important, and a health education programme can be introduced that promotes early diagnosis and the acceptability of any treatment offered. In 1982, 33% of men and 23% of women over 60 years of age were current smokers.[13] When an elderly patient is dying at home the primary care team needs all its skills. They can offer complete care when the patient may need them most and can continue to support the bereaved. Hospice care in some areas extends into the community and can be supplementary.

The future

The identification of the elderly in general practice is essential for a preventive programme, and it is to be hoped that family practitioner committees will provide geriatric age-sex registers as a regular service. A small number of computer systems have been installed in family practitioner committee offices. Microcomputers are arriving in general practices, and the small numbers are being boosted by the recent Department of Health and Social Security scheme. Transport for the elderly is still difficult, and improvement is imperative. Easier communication by provision of more telephones is also needed. The provision of more day centres and day hospitals will enable the care of the elderly in general practice to continue at a high standard.

[1] Department of Health and Social Security. *On the state of the public health for the year 1982*. London: HMSO, 1983.
[2] Hodes C. Geriatric screening and care in group practice. *J R Coll Gen Pract* 1971; **31**: 469.
[3] Williams EI, *et al*. Sociomedical study of patients over 75 in general practice. *Br Med J* 1972; ii: 445.
[4] Royal College of General Practice. Working Party on Prevention. *Prevention of arterial disease in general practice*. London: Royal College of General Practice, 1981.
[5] Williams P, Clare A. Management of psychosocial disorder in general practice. In: *Psychosocial disorders in general practice*. London: Academic Press, 1979.
[6] Harte JD. Preparing for retirement. *J R Coll Gen Pract* 1972; **22**: 612.
[7] Office of Population Censuses and Surveys. Social Survey Division. *The general household survey 1979*. London: HMSO, 1981.
[8] Weed LL. *Medical records, medical education and patient care*. Ohio: Cleveland, 1971.
[9] Williamson J, *et al*. Old people at home: their unreported needs. *Lancet* 1964; i: 1117.
[10] Lowther CP, MacLeod, RDM, Williamson J. Evaluation of early diagnostic services for the elderly. *Br Med J* 1970; **3**: 275
[11] Hodes C. The structure and function of a file of patient health data in general practice. *J R Coll Gen Pract* 1968; **15**: 286.
[12] Forbes JA. Locating the elderly in general practice. *Br Med J* 1969; ii: 46.
[13] Central Statistical Office. *Social trends*. London: HMSO, 1984.
[14] Royal College of General Practice, Office of Population Censuses and Surveys, Department of Health and Social Security. *Morbidity statistics from general practice 1971–72. Second national survey*. London: HMSO, 1979.

Role of day hospitals in the care of the elderly

J C BROCKLEHURST

Geriatric medicine initiated an early form of progressive patient care in hospital – through acute admission ward, to rehabilitation ward, and continuing care ward. The geriatric day hospital is a logical extension of this system and forms a bridge between the hospital and the community. The ever increasing numbers and proportion of elderly people, particularly the very old, in our society inevitably increase the incidence of disabling disease. The provision of day care for the treatment and support of elderly disabled people has been an attempt, attended with a good deal of success, to prevent the admission to hospital of more and more of these old people.

Social day care

Day care for the elderly includes a wide variety of social and hospital provisions, which must be clearly distinguished. Social day care is provided either by local authorities or by voluntary organisations (for example, Age Concern organisations) – or occasionally by thoughtful employers. Social day care itself offers a whole spectrum of facilities.[1] Anderson's definition of social day care is as follows: "Clubs and social centres exist for all old people, to increase social contact and to give scope and facilities for new pursuits in retirement."

Several main types of day care are now available.[2] Day care centres, most usually instituted by local authorities, provide a substantial amount of personal care to at least a small proportion of clients. Referral is usually through general practitioners or social workers. There is a wide range of services, including bathing, chiropody, meals, and provision of low priced foods.

Both these types of social day centres may be provided by local authorities under the 1968 Health Services and Public Health Act and both require transport to bring the clients to them.

Social centres or social clubs come in many varieties: some are open seven days a week, others only one half day a fortnight. They usually have a regular membership and are often organised by the retired people themselves. Shelters (rest centre or drop in) may be provided by local communities or employers and serve simply as a communal meeting place that elderly people may use as they wish.

Communal rooms in sheltered housing and other housing schemes clearly offer a great opportunity for day care, in which both residents in the sheltered housing and other people living in the area may join together. A most important development for the future will be the provision of a restaurant so that residents in sheltered housing may have at least one communal cooked meal a day, at which they may be joined by elderly people from the local community.

Lunch clubs are an important and desirable alternative to meals on wheels. Work centres may be provided either by the local authority, commercial organisations, or voluntary bodies. Essentially, retired people come here to engage in productive work for which they are paid. This has, of course, very important social and emotional advantages.

These various types of social day care available at present must be clearly distinguished from the geriatric day hospital.

Day hospitals

Day hospitals are part of the hospital service and are generally situated within a district general hospital in close relation to the geriatric rehabilitation department.[2,3] In many cases day hospital and geriatric rehabilitation department share the same premises and facilities. This is a particularly desirable concept, which allows patients who have been undergoing rehabilitation to return to their homes and yet have the security of a continuing contact with the hospital, and so with their therapists, until they are firmly settled back at home. Though day hospitals have many uses other than this, this is one of the most important and one which guards against waste of hospital resources.

The concept of a geriatric day hospital must now be extended to include the psychogeriatric day hospital. It is part of the clearly defined policy of the Department of Health and Social Security to provide two places per 1000 people over 65 for geriatric day hospital care and an additional two places per 1000 people over 65 for psychogeriatric day hospital care. The psychogeriatric day hospital may be established adjoining the geriatric day hospital and share several facilities. Alternatively, and hitherto more commonly, it may be set up within a psychiatric hospital, though in future, of course, these will be replaced. A further possibility is that the psychogeriatric day hospital may be situated within the community hospital or general practitioner hospital, particularly in rural areas.[4]

Development

Geriatric day hospitals first developed from occupational therapy departments. The first purpose built geriatric day hospital was opened in Oxford at Cowley Road Hospital, and this has served as the model for subsequent development. The day hospital at Oxford was opened in 1958, and by the end of 1970 there were 120 geriatric day hospitals in the UK. Now most geriatric departments include a day hospital, and increasingly purpose built day hospitals are superseding adaptations of various other hospital premises.

Work

Elderly patients come to a day hospital for one of four main reasons: rehabilitation; maintenance treatment; medical or nursing investigation; or social care.

Rehabilitation is an important part of geriatric practice since so often the problem is one of physical disability: there is a prospect of improvement, though often not of recovery. It is helpful to see rehabilitation as a finite process to which there is usually an end – reached when the patient achieves his maximum degree of independence.

Maintenance treatment is important in old age since having once achieved maximum independence many elderly people will deteriorate slowly (and sometimes quite rapidly) once they are cut off from the stimulus of the geriatric rehabilitation department. Much important and laborious work can thereby be undone, particularly if relatives are overprotective or the old person is poorly motivated. Day hospital attendance once a week perhaps for an indefinite period often ensures that the state of independence achieved is maintained.

Medical and nursing procedures in the day hospital form a very variable part of current geriatric practice. In a few departments great stress is laid on these; in most some use is made of the day hospital for procedures such as sternal marrow punctures, the supervision and treatment of faecal incontinence, glucose tolerance tests, etc. On the other hand, obviously it is not appropriate to bring elderly people up to a day hospital simply to carry out procedures that might equally well be done by the district nurse or the family doctor in the patient's home. Some geriatric departments use the day hospital also as the setting for their outpatient clinic.

The distinction between social day care and the geriatric day hospital has already been emphasised, but a few elderly people are so physically disabled as to be unsuitable for social day centres and yet have needs for companionship and relief of their isolation. Its nursing care makes a geriatric day hospital the appropriate place for such patients. Another, occasional, aspect of social care is when a disabled elderly patient may be discharged home from hospital and looked after at night and at the weekend, but when the relative on whom he depends has to work. Discharge may then be possible only if day hospital attendance can be arranged. The most important social aspect of the day hospital, however, is to provide relief for relatives caring for heavily dependent old people. This may be linked with intermittent patient care ("shared care") as a means of maintaining such elderly patients as long as possible in their own homes.

Patients

In a national survey of day hospitals Brocklehurst and Tucker[3] found that consultant geriatricians placed most importance on rehabilitation and maintenance (46% and 38% of respondents). Of patients actually attending 30 day hospitals, however, rather fewer were coming for these two reasons (43% for rehabilitation and 21% for maintenance). Nineteen per cent were attending for nursing care and 17% for social care. The majority attended one or two days weekly (47% one day and 41% two days). The larger number of patients were referred by their general practitioners (61% of 456 new referrals) and accepted principally by way of a domiciliary consultation or outpatient clinic attendance. The remainder came immediately after discharge from hospital (28% from geriatric wards, 9% from other wards). Most of the patients (82%) were aged between 65 and 85, while a small number (13%) were older than 85 years. The principal diagnosis among those attending was stroke (37%), followed by arthritis (22%).

Staff

The day hospital should be regarded as a ward within the hospital – in fact, Andrews has suggested that it should be called a day ward rather than a day hospital. This emphasises that staffing should be on similar levels to that of an inpatient ward and that management should be along similar lines. The day hospital is generally in the charge of the consultant geriatrician and consists of three main departments – nursing, physiotherapy, and occupational therapy – with a smaller involvement of speech therapists, social workers, volunteers, and administrators. A doctor must attend daily to maintain records and to initiate investigation and treatment of patients. There should also be a case conference of the whole medical, social, and therapeutic team at least once weekly to review the patients' progress. To be dynamic a day hospital must be continually discharging and accepting new patients, and there should never be a waiting list. It is a great advantage if there are clear pathways between the day hospital and the various social day care facilities so that those who no longer need the therapeutic aspect of day care may continue to enjoy its social benefit.

Advantages

The advantages of the geriatric day hospital lie first in allowing the treatment of many elderly people without hospital admission, particularly when outpatient attendance at a physiotherapy department would be unsuitable. The need is for a continuing therapeutic environment where the pace is slower but activity continues throughout most of the day. The day hospital also allows the earlier discharge of patients and their subsequent supervision until they are safely settled at home. Another advantage is that the hours are attractive to staff and recruitment of suitable staff is often easier than to the inpatient wards.

Problems

Day hospitals are not without their problems. Probably the greatest of these lies in the provision of ambulance transport. It is exceptional for any patient needing day hospital treatment to be able to come independently. A few can be brought by relatives in cars, and in the occasional area taxis are hired for this purpose, but generally day hospitals must depend on the ambulance service for the delivery and returning home of their patients. This requires special and appropriate transport – for example, a vehicle with eight to 10 seats with a hydraulic or other lift, good visibility for the passengers, safe seating, and good heating. Such a vehicle is likely to take between an hour and an hour and a half to collect its complement of patients, and so those collected first may well spend upwards of an hour in the vehicle. For most of them this is no hardship provided that the vehicle is appropriate, since it is likely to be the only time that they get out of their own homes.

It is essential that ambulances should bring patients to the day hospital and take them home according to a prearranged timetable and that vehicles are not used that are apt to be diverted for other purposes. The whole professional team in the day hospital awaits the arrival of the patients, and if ambulance services are erratic there is an enormous waste of these professional resources. It is equally frustrating for the old person sitting for two or three hours awaiting the ambulance's arrival. Furthermore, patients coming to day hospitals are often relying on this as their only source of food that day, and perhaps of heating and other care. If the ambulance does not collect them they may suffer great hardship, as was shown in a survey of the effect of industrial action by the ambulance service on day hospital patients.[5]

Finally, what of the future? The day hospital is now firmly established, and almost every geriatric department now has one as an essential part of its service. There may be an increase of specialisation within day hospitals, some developing more as day wards for medical and nursing treatment, others becoming the local stroke rehabilitation unit or orthopaedic rehabilitation unit for elderly people. Possibly some smaller day hospitals may be set up in association with community hospitals, where the emphasis will be on maintenance and social treatment. The day hospital serves as an excellent focus bringing together community medical care (the general practitioner team) and the geriatric hospital team. The day hospital is in many ways a shop window for the geriatric service, and a good one undoubtedly adds immeasurably to the morale of the whole geriatric department.

[1] Anderson DC. *Report on leisure and day care facilities for the old.* London: Age Concern, 1972.

[2] Carter J. *Day services for adults.* London: Allen and Unwin, 1981. (National Institute of Social Services Library No 40.)

[3] Brocklehurst JC, Tucker JS. *Progress in geriatric day care.* London: King Edward's Hospital Fund for London, 1980.

[4] Arie T. Day care and geriatric psychiatry. *Gerontologia Clinica* 1975; **17**: 31–9.

[5] Andrews J, Fairley A, Hyland M. A geriatric day ward in an English hospital. *J Am Geriatrics Soc* 1970; **18**: 378–86.

[6] Prinsley DN. Effects of industrial action by the ambulance service on day hospital patients. *Br Med J* 1971; iii: 170–1.

Skeletal disease in the elderly

J T LEEMING

Prevalence

In this chapter patients over 75 will generally be under consideration, though in calculating prevalence it is convenient to use the age of 65. Mention will be made of five disorders: (a) osteoporosis; (b) Paget's disease; (c) osteomalacia; (d) malignant disease, including multiple myeloma; and (e) medical aspects of fractured neck of femur.

It is important to consider the frequency with which these conditions are likely to occur in an average general practice. A general practitioner's list of 3000 patients will be assumed to have 420 patients over the age of 65 (255 women and 165 men). Geriatric departments serving a population of 240 000 and admitting 1000 a year will be assumed to serve 80 general practitioners.

Osteoporosis, with a susceptibility to fracture, affects 25% of women over the age of 65, and men are probably affected a quarter as frequently as women. The prevalence of Paget's disease rises to 10% by the age of 90, so a prevalence of 6% will be assumed for those over 65. Men are affected more often than women. Osteomalacia, mostly occurring in women, is found in between 1% and 4% of geriatric hospital admissions, the higher figure in Glasgow and the lower figure in the south of England. The prevalence of femoral neck fracture is found to be two per 1000 during the period 65 to 74, nine per 1000 in the age group 75 to 84, and 25 per 1000 in those aged 85 and over.

Using these figures and assumptions I have calculated that a general practitioner with a list of 3000 will have on his list 72 patients with osteoporosis (64 women and eight men) and 25 patients with Paget's disease (about 15 men and 10 women) and that he will see a case of osteomalacia once every two to eight years. The prevalence of malignant disease has not been calculated

Incidence, preventability, treatability, and seriousness if not treated of various conditions

Incidence	Preventability	Treatability	Seriousness if not treated
Osteoporosis + + +	Osteomalacia + + +	Osteomalacia + + +	Malignancy + + +
Paget's + +	Osteoporosis ±	Paget's + +	Osteomalacia + +
Osteomalacia ±	Paget's ○	Malignancy +	Osteoporosis +
Malignancy ±	Malignancy ○	Osteoporosis ±	Paget's ±

○ − + + + = rough guide to relative importance of diseases under each heading.

but will not be high. Two or three cases of fractured neck of femur are likely to occur each year.

In the table the prevalence of the first four conditions is compared and they are placed very broadly in order with regard to preventability, treatability, and seriousness if untreated.

The less common conditions merit more emphasis than their prevalence would suggest because they can be treated and cause more trouble if untreated; osteomalacia can be prevented and so may osteoporosis in a more limited sense. All four conditions lead to bones being fractured by relatively minor trauma so that this is not a useful way of differentiating them. The fact that fractures may easily occur in the elderly should constantly be borne in mind because the absence of severe trauma and the presence of other diseases make it easy to overlook them. Thus the patient with a hemiplegia may have a fractured neck of femur on the same side, the lady with painful arthritis of the hips may fracture the neck of the femur, and the patient with cracked and painful ribs due to osteomalacia may also have angina and may be too anxious or confused to give a clear description. Fractured neck of femur is considered from an orthopaedic point of view in a later chapter. Taking a long view, however, it is as much of a medical as a surgical problem, and the medical factors will be briefly outlined.

Osteoporosis

Though osteoporosis is, broadly speaking, a benign disorder, it may exact a considerable price in terms of episodic morbidity, the consequences becoming more serious with increasing age. In this condition there is a generalised loss of bone, the bone which remains being normal. The serum calcium, phosphorus, and alkaline phosphatase levels are not affected, and there are no symptoms or signs until structural failure occurs. The amount of bone in the skeleton increases until the age of 20 to 25, after which it very slowly declines. Women accumulate less bone than men and tend to lose it more quickly. Structural failure usually begins in women over the age of 50 and in men over the age of about 65. It shows itself in a loss of height and thoracic kyphosis due to narrowing of the vertebral bodies and a wedge shaped deformity of the thoracic vertebrae. The lower ribs sink towards the iliac crest. Fractures occur in the lower forearm in women over the age of 50 and in the neck of the femur in both sexes over the age of 70. Compression fractures occur from time to time in the lower thoracic and lumbar vertebrae, which characteristically produce severe localised backache that clears up in three to four weeks. Neurological sequelae rarely if ever occur. Probably vertebral fractures are often not recognised at the time. Recognition is made more difficult by the fact that only a minority of cases of backache can be traced to osteoporosis.[1]

Bed rest has repeatedly been shown to lead to a negative calcium balance, and hypercalciuria persists even if the legs are exercised in bed. There is evidence that resumption of mobility may lead to the restoration of bone lost during bed rest, and the value of exercise is borne out by studies showing that athletes have denser bones than non-athletes and that less strenuous exercise may be of value.[2] The long term therapeutic administration of corticosteroids is well known to induce osteoporosis, trabecular bone in the spine and ribs being mainly affected.[3]

Substances that have been considered in the treatment of osteoporosis can be divided into those that prevent bone loss – for example, calcium, oestrogen, calcitonin and the thiazide diuretics, and those that may restore skeletal mass by stimulating bone formation, such as fluoride, growth hormone, and the human synthetic parathyroid hormone fragment HPTH (1–34).[4] Oestrogens have been found to prevent postmenopausal bone loss. In one prospective study various combinations of calcium, oestrogen, and fluoride were found to reduce the rate of vertebral fracture, the most striking effect being found when all three substances were given.[5] A retrospective inquiry, comparing women who had taken oestrogens for six years or longer with a group who had not taken them, found the risk of fracture of the hip or lower forearm to be 50 % to 60 % lower in the oestrogen group.[6] Unfortunately there are risks from side effects or other practical difficulties in giving most of these substances. A recent review provides an excellent critique of present knowledge on treatment regimens.[7]

Taking an adequate amount of calcium and exercise would seem to be the least toxic measure, and the thiazide diuretics, which have been shown to cause calcium retention,[8] may be worth bearing in mind.

To prevent excessive bone loss periods of bed rest should be kept as short as possible throughout life. If adrenocortical steroids have to be given their effect in increasing osteoporosis must be borne in mind. When fractures occur due to osteoporosis they should be treated promptly and analgesics prescribed to permit a speedy return to normal activity. Temporary admission to hospital may be indicated to achieve quicker mobilisation. Attention to the other medical and social conditions so often present in old people will help to increase mobility and also reduce the likelihood of falls in the future. Home conditions should be investigated and hazards removed or alleviated whenever possible. A reasonable amount of exercise should be encouraged. Diet should be adequate and varied, especially with regard to calcium. A daily pint of milk would provide at least half of the necessary calcium intake.

Paget's disease

There is evidence of geographical, racial, and familial variation in the incidence of this disorder.[9] In a study of radiological prevalence in 14 towns in England and Wales a somewhat higher prevalence was found in the Preston, Bolton, and Blackburn area than elsewhere.[10] Osteoclasts seem to be the bone cells involved, and, although the cause is not known, recent studies have shown cytoplasmic and nuclear inclusion bodies that suggest that the disease may be due to a slow virus infection.[11]

The skeleton is affected in a patchy, asymmetrical manner. Most commonly affected are the pelvis, lumbar spine, femur, tibia, skull, and clavicle. At the affected sites there is a greatly increased bone turnover. The new bone is spongy and disorganised, leading to expansion and deformity, and gross bowing may occur in the femur and tibia. It is a disease that may have phases of activity and inactivity. During active phases the affected bone is warm to the touch and the serum alkaline phosphatase activity may be grossly raised. The serum calcium and phosphorus concentrations are usually normal. The increased circulation through the affected bone may sometimes precipitate or exacerbate heart failure, but this seems to happen very little in the elderly. Pain in the affected bone may be severe, but this also is uncommon in my experience. Practical problems can result from gross deformities and from nerve deafness due to compression of the eighth nerve by the enlarged bone. Paget's disease varies enormously in extent, sometimes only one clavicle being affected. In rare instances when the spine is affected neurological effects such as paraplegia may be produced.

Most cases are asymptomatic and should be given no treatment.

81

Some patients develop bone pain that is usually best controlled by simple analgesics. More specific drugs should be reserved for the following situations, and only given under close supervision: severe bone pain that is unresponsive to analgesics and unlikely to be due to concomitant osteoarthritis; neurological compression problems such as paraplegia due to spinal involvement; before and after orthopaedic surgery; and in rare instances where immobilisation leads to hypercalcaemia.[12] The drugs currently in use are calcitonin, which reduces the abnormally high turnover of bone cells and may lead to some remodelling of the bone,[13] and the diphosphonates, which suppress the numbers and activity of the osteoclasts.[12] Calcitonin rarely produces serious side effects but has to be injected subcutaneously. Diphosphonate is taken by mouth two hours before meals, but a recent paper showed a tendency to increased osteoid formation at sites of the disease with an increased risk of fracture of weight bearing bones, even with low dosage.[14] For either drug to be continued, there should be some evidence of pain reduction within three months, with a fall in the serum alkaline phosphatase activity. Both drugs are usually given for about six months at a time. There is some evidence that they may be combined with advantage.[12] After calcitonin improvement may be maintained for six to 12 months and after diphosphonate treatment for up to two or three years. Improved diphosphonate derivatives may become available in the next few years.[12] A suggested dose of salmon calcitonin (salcatonin) is 200 units subcutaneously two or three times a week and for the diphosphonate disodium etidronate 400 mg daily to be taken two hours before a meal.

Osteomalacia

Osteomalacia is characterised histologically by failure of newly formed bone (osteoid) to calcify. The serum calcium and phosphorus concentrations are often, though not invariably, reduced and the serum alkaline phosphatase activity is raised in 80% of cases. Iliac crest bone biopsy, which can be performed using a local anaesthetic, is the most reliable single method of diagnosis.

Weakness of the proximal limb muscles is a major manifestation and leads to difficulty lifting the feet over kerbstones and ultimately to the necessity of going up and downstairs on all fours. The gait may be rolling or "waddling" in character. This weakness can often be shown by formal neurological examination in young subjects, but in old patients the presence of multiple pathology usually prevents a convincing display. Difficulty in walking or an inability to walk is a leading symptom, however, and myopathy can be inferred from this. Bone pain – especially in the back, thighs, shoulder region, or ribs is usually present – and the bones may be tender. The pain is worse on muscular effort. Quite often, especially in those patients seen in geriatric departments, the pain is vague and undramatic. Characteristically it occurs in several of the above sites. Fractures of the ribs are more common in osteomalacia than in osteoporosis, and possibly their significance has sometimes been underestimated. The clinical features were reviewed by Chalmers.[15]

Osteomalacia is more common after partial gastrectomy, in patients on phenobarbitone and other anticonvulsants, and where there is intestinal malabsorption. It is now realised that vitamin D deficiency is mainly due to reduced exposure to ultraviolet light even in people with adjuvant factors such as antiepileptic therapy, steatorrhoea, and liver disease.[16,17] Such patients often get very little exposure to sunshine because of their reduced mobility or institutionalisation. The usual diet contains very little vitamin D. Blood concentrations of 25 hydroxyvitamin D have been repeatedly shown to be higher in the summer months than in the winter months, and small amounts of exposure to ultraviolet light are effective in restoring low levels to normal.[18] Osteomalacia occurs more often in the housebound elderly.[19]

When venous blood is taken to support the diagnosis the patient should be fasting, and it is important to use only the minimum tourniquet pressure. The serum proteins and blood urea should be estimated at the same time because a reduction of the albumin level will lead to a lowering of serum calcium and a raised urea concentration will cause a rise in the serum phosphorus. It is worth checking the blood count at the same time to exclude anaemia; x ray films of the chest, lumbar spine, and pelvis are helpful, partly to exclude Paget's disease as the cause for a raised serum alkaline phosphatase activity and partly because the presence of incomplete fractures (Looser's zones) in the pubic rami, femoral neck, axillary border of scapula, or upper end of the humerus is virtual proof of the diagnosis. Unfortunately they are seen in only a minority of cases. As it is curable osteomalacia should be excluded in any old person who is bedfast or having difficulty getting about without obvious cause, or when the above symptoms are present.

Osteomalacia is often difficult to diagnose in hospital without bone biopsy. It is even more difficult in general practice where it occurs much less frequently. The best plan, therefore, is to refer suspected patients to hospital for further consideration. Once diagnosed the condition is not difficult to treat. A suggested scheme is to give calciferol 50 000 units (1.25 mg) daily for two weeks followed by tablets of calcium and vitamin D (BPC) in a dose of one tablet twice daily for 12 months. It is important not to prolong treatment with the larger dose of calciferol, which would be likely to produce hypercalcaemia followed by renal failure.

Bone pain usually clears and the serum calcium and phosphorus return to normal within two weeks, but it may be six to eight months before the serum alkaline phosphatase activity falls to within normal limits. When treatment is begun the serum alkaline phosphatase activity often rises temporarily. In young people muscle weakness recovers within a week or two, but in the elderly this may take as much as a month or two because of the reduced general fitness and presence of other disorders particularly arthritis.

Regular prophylaxis

To prevent a recurrence of osteomalacia and to prevent its development in housebound patients over the age of 75 it is logical to give regular prophylactic vitamin D, such as tablets of calcium with vitamin D (BPC), which contain 500 units (12.5 μg) of vitamin D, or vitamin A and D capsules (BPC), which contain 400 units (10 μg), in a dose of one tablet or capsule daily for three or four months in the winter. It has been shown that one tablet of calcium with vitamin D given daily will restore lower concentrations of plasma 25 hydroxyvitamin D to normal in two months.[20] Another method of prophylaxis might be to give a big dose, such as 2.5 mg of calciferol, once a year.[21] Even small amounts of exposure to the sun are beneficial and should be encouraged.

It is worth noting that osteomalacia may occur in patients with other more obvious bone disorders. Thus I have seen bone pain in a patient with breast metastases, and backache in a patient with Paget's disease, clear up when vitamin D was given. The serum phosphorus concentration was initially low in both patients. A therapeutic trial of vitamin D (for example, 50 000 units daily for not more than a week or two) is well justified in this situation.

Malignant disease

Multiple myeloma is not rare in hospital practice. Bone pain in one or more sites, especially the back, is a common presentation, and pathological fractures may occur. The serum calcium concentration may be normal or raised; the serum phosphorus and alkaline phosphatase concentrations are normal. The x ray films may show clear cut translucent areas, which may give a "lead shot" appearance in a lateral view of the skull. In other cases a generalised osteoporosis is the only bone change seen. Anaemia and renal failure may be complications, and Bence Jones protein may be found in the urine. The erythrocyte sedimentation rate is usually high and the serum globulin concentration considerably raised, with an abnormal peak on electrophoresis.

A remission for a year or two may often be induced by chemotherapy with, for example, a combination of melphalan and prednisone,[22] but old people withstand chemotherapy less well, and it is especially important in this age group to withhold treatment unless there are symptoms due to anaemia, bone lesions, hypercalcaemia, or renal impairment.[23] Radiotherapy is effective for localised severe bone pain.

Bony metastases from carcinoma of the prostate and carcinoma of the breast may cause much pain and disability. To make the diagnosis and to determine the extent of bony involvement a combination of radiography and isotope bone scanning is helpful. The serum alkaline phosphatase activity is likely to be raised, and sometimes the serum calcium concentration is also high. If carcinoma of the prostate is the cause there is often a rise of the serum acid phosphatase activity. Initially a good response may be expected to tamoxifen 10 mg orally twice daily in 34% of patients with breast metastases[24] and to oestrogens, such as diethyl stilboestrol 2 to 5 mg daily, in 70–80% of patients with prostatic metastases.[25] In both cases relapse usually occurs within a year or two.

Fracture of the femoral neck

The incidence of fractured neck of femur increases steeply with increasing age; however, the increase in incidence in the past 15 years has greatly exceeded the increase in the numbers of the very old, which account for only a third of the increase.[26] The reasons for this recent disproportionate rise in the frequency of fracture are not known, but it has been suggested that one factor may be a general decrease in the mobility of old people.[27] Most hip fractures occur indoors and are not due to slipping outside on ice and snow as was previously thought. The prognosis for restoration of mobility after treatment of the fracture depends mainly on the associated medical conditions present.

Conditions significantly related to fracture of the femoral neck include osteoporosis, osteomalacia, dementia, an above average frequency of falling, pyramidal tract abnormalities, poor eyesight, and reduced body weight.[28,29] In one series of hospital patients 46 out of 50 had concurrent medical problems – dementia, heart failure, vertebrobasilar ischaemia and drop attacks, bronchitis and emphysema, and hemiparesis being the most frequent.[30] In the same series complications while in hospital were, in descending order of frequency, incontinence of urine, incontinence of faeces, pressure sores, and deep vein thrombosis.

A recent study found that the increase in incidence of fracture in cold weather was mainly due to an increased incidence in very thin old people while indoors.[31] In most of these patients the core temperature was less than 35 °C on admission, whereas well nourished patients were usually normothermic. The authors suggest that the mild hypothermia led to poorer coordination, which predisposed to accidental trauma. In a second study the same authors found that thinner patients had a lower voluntary food intake, higher mortality, and a longer rehabilitation time.[32] Dietary supplementation shortened both rehabilitation time and hospital stay.

Clearly more work is needed to determine the reasons for the recent increase of femoral fracture and the importance of nutritional factors. In the meantime, there is much that general practitioners can do to prevent fracture by treating or seeking further advice on the associated conditions mentioned. A good place to start would be to see whether eyesight can be improved and whether lighting in the house is adequate; old people need lighting of twice the intensity needed by younger people. Once the patient is in hospital the need for cooperation between physicians and surgeons is self evident.

[1] Adams P, Davies GT, Sweetnam P. Osteoporosis and the effects of ageing on bone mass in elderly men and women. *Q J Med* 1970; **39**: 601–15.

[2] Anonymous. Osteoporosis and activity. *Lancet* 1983; i: 1365–6.

[3] Baylink DJ. Glucocorticoid-induced osteoporosis *N Engl J Med* 1983; **309**: 306–8.

[4] Anonymous. Treatment of osteoporosis. *Br Med J* 1978; i: 1303–4.

[5] Riggs BL, Seeman E, Hodgson SF, *et al.* Effect of the fluoride/calcium regimen on vertebral fracture occurrence in postmenopausal osteoporosis. *N Engl J Med* 1982; **306**: 446–50.

[6] Weiss NS, Ure CL, Ballard JH, *et al.* Decreased risk of fractures of the hip and lower forearm with postmenopausal use of estrogen. *N Engl J Med* 1980; **303**: 1195–8.

[7] Kanis JA. Treatment of osteoporotic fracture. *Lancet* 1984; i: 27–32.

[8] Wasnich RD, Benfante RJ, Yano K, *et al.* Thiazide effect on the mineral content of bone. *N Engl J Med* 1983; **309**: 344–7.

[9] Anonymous. Paget's disease of bone. *Br Med J* 1977; i: 1427–8.

[10] Barker DJP, Clough PWL, Guyer PB, *et al.* Paget's disease of bone in 14 British towns. *Br Med J* 1977; i: 1181.

[11] Anonymous. Viruses and Paget's disease of bone. *Lancet* 1982; ii: 1198–9.

[12] Hosking DJ. Paget's disease of bone. *Br Med J* 1981; **283**: 686–8.

[13] Evans IMA. Calcitonin treatment of Paget's disease. *Lancet* 1979; ii: 1232–3.

[14] Boyce BF, Fogelman I, Ralston S, *et al.* Focal osteomalacia due to low-dose diphosphonate therapy in Paget's disease. *Lancet* 1984; i: 821–4.

[15] Chalmers J. Osteomalacia: a review of 93 cases. *Journal of the Royal College of Surgeons of Edinburgh* 1968; **13**: 255–75.

[16] Fraser DR. The physiological economy of vitamin D. *Lancet* 1983; i: 969–72.
[17] Anonymous. Hepatic osteomalacia and vitamin D. *Lancet* 1982; i: 943–4.
[18] Snell AP, MacLennan WJ, Hamilton JC. Ultra-violet irradiation and 25 – hydroxy-vitamin D levels in sick old people. *Age Ageing* 1978; 7: 225–8.
[19] Webster SGP, Leeming JT, Wilkinson EM. The causes of osteomalacia in the elderly. *Age Ageing* 1976; 5: 119–22.
[20] MacLennan WJ, Hamilton JC. Vitamin D supplements and 25 – hydroxy vitamin D concentrations in the elderly. *Br Med J* 1977; ii: 859–61.
[21] Stephens WP, Berry JL, Klimiuk PS, *et al*. Annual high-dose vitamin D prophylaxis in Asian immigrants. *Lancet* 1981; ii: 1199–201.
[22] McIntyre OR. Current concepts in cancer: multiple myeloma. *N Engl J Med* 1979; **301**: 193–6.
[23] Kyle RA, Greipp PR. Smoldering multiple myeloma. *N Engl J Med* 1980; **302**; 1347–9.
[24] Smith IE, Harris AL, Morgan M, *et al*. Tamoxifen versus aminoglutethimide in advanced breast carcinoma: a randomised cross-over trial. *Br Med J* 1981; **283**: 1432–4.
[25] Klein LA. Medical progress: prostatic carcinoma. *N Engl J Med* 1979; **300**: 824–33.
[26] Lewis AF. Fracture of neck of the femur: changing indicence. *Br Med J* 1981; **283**: 1217–20.
[27] Wallace WA. The increasing incidence of fractures of the proximal femur: an orthopaedic epidemic. *Lancet* 1983; i: 1413.
[28] Brocklehurst JC, Exton-Smith AN, Lempert-Barber SM, *et al*. Fracture of the femur in old age: a two-centre study of associated clinical factors and the cause of the fall. *Age Ageing* 1978; 7: 7–15.
[29] Wootton R, Bryson E, Elsasser U, *et al*. Risk factors for fractured neck of femur in the elderly. *Age Ageing* 1982; **11**: 160–8.
[30] Campbell AJ. Femoral neck fractures in elderly women: a prospective study. *Age Ageing* 1976; 5: 102–9.
[31] Bastow MD, Rawlings J, Allison SP. Undernutrition, hypothermia, and injury in elderly women with fractured femur: an injury response to altered metabolism? *Lancet* 1983; i: 143–6.
[32] Bastow MD, Rawlings J, Allison SP. Benefits of supplementary tube feeding after fractured neck of femur: a randomised controlled trial. *Br Med J* 1983; **287**: 1589–92.

Accidental hypothermia

A N EXTON-SMITH

It is generally considered that a hypothermic state exists when the deep body temperature falls below an arbitrarily defined limit of 35 °C. The term accidental hypothermia is used to imply that the lowering of the body temperature is unintentional and it has to be distinguished from hypothermia induced for the purposes of medical or surgical treatment.

Incidence

The British Medical Association's committee on accidental hypothermia in the elderly,[1] after reviewing the descriptions of cases published in Britain up to the early 1960s, concluded that there was no accurate information on the incidence of the condition. The hospital reports indicated that very few cases were recognised before admission and elderly people with hypothermia suffered a high mortality. Death resulted from the often serious nature of the underlying disease as well as from the effects of hypothermia itself.

The Registrar General's returns of death certificates indicate that only about 100 fatal cases are reported annually.[2] These figures are at variance with those reported in the survey conducted by the Royal College of Physicians.[3] Ten hospital groups cooperated in the investigation, and during the three months 1 February to 30 April 1965 it was found that 126 patients had rectal temperatures of 35 °C or less on admission, representing 0.68 % of all admissions. It was estimated that there could have been 9000 patients admitted to hospitals in England and Wales with hypothermia during the three winter months and 42 % of these patients were over the age of 65. The true incidence is probably much higher than this, especially among the elderly, since the survey did not include those patients treated at home, in many of whom hypothermia passes unrecognised.

Relations between body temperature and environmental conditions

The results of the first large scale national survey of body temperatures of old people in Great Britain living at home were reported by Fox *et al* in 1973.[2] The investigation was based on measurements made on 1020 people of 65 and over during the first three months of 1972. In 754 cases (75%) the room temperatures of the old people were at or below 18.3 °C (65 °F) – the minimum recommended by the Parker Morris report on council housing – and in 10% the morning living room temperatures were very cold, at or below 12.0 °C. The deep body temperatures in the morning and evening were measured by the Uritemp technique. In about 10% of subjects the deep body temperatures were below 35.5 °C (low group), and these were considered to be at risk of developing hypothermia. In comparison with a normal group (36.0 °C and above), not only were they less successful in conserving body heat, as shown by their inability to maintain an adequate core-shell temperature gradient; they also had a proportionately lower body heat content. The high prevalence of low room temperatures and of low body temperatures in the morning clearly indicated the need for measures to protect the individual from cold exposure at night. Disturbingly many individuals whose temperatures were in the low group were already receiving supplementary benefits, and yet only 3% of these pensioners were receiving an extra fuel allowance.

Aetiology

As is the case for many disorders in old age, multiple aetiological factors are responsible. This applies to accidental hypothermia in the elderly and the main factors can be grouped under five headings

● Exposure to cold
● Impaired thermoregulation
● Impaired shivering thermogenesis
● Impaired temperature perception
● Diseases and drugs

Exposure to cold

Exposure to cold is an overriding cause, and there is a clear relation between the incidence of accidental hypothermia and a low environmental temperature. A common story is of an old person who falls after attempting to get out of bed at night; he remains on the floor for several hours, often partly clad, and is discovered only the next day by a neighbour or a home help. Thus probably the exposure is longer when the old person lives alone and is socially isolated. Very many cases, however, occur with lesser degrees of exposure, while the old person is in bed at night apparently well covered. In these instances insufficient body heat is being generated, so that even good external insulation is ineffective.

Impaired thermoregulation

The high incidence of accidental hypothermia in old people can mainly be accounted for by a physiological decline in thermoregulatory function, which has been shown in both cross sectional and longitudinal studies.[2,4] In many old people the normal core–shell temperature difference of 4.5° to 5.0 °C cannot be maintained owing to impaired vasoconstriction in response to cold.

Impaired shivering thermogenesis

Collins et al have compared the metabolic response to cooling in healthy elderly subjects and young control subjects using a body cooling unit.[5] Shivering was absent or less intense in the older group, and the increase in metabolic heat production was significantly less than in the young controls.

Impaired thermal perception

Many old people have a diminished sensitivity to cold. Tests of digital thermosensation[6] show that young people can perceive mean temperature differences of about 0.8 °C whereas elderly subjects can discriminate only between mean temperature differences of 2.5 °C, and some are unable to perceive differences of 5 °C or more. It is likely that a lesser sensitivity to cold is one of the reasons for the relatively large number of old people who appear to be able to tolerate cold conditions without discomfort. Nevertheless, they may be at risk of overtaxing the heat conserving capacity of a failing thermoregulatory system.

Diseases and drugs

In addition to this age related impairment of physiological functions the most severe cases of hypothermia in patients admitted to hospital have some underlying clinical condition. Almost any serious disorder may cause hypothermia, but those commonly found are:

Endocrine disorders – myxoedema and hypopituitarism in which the metabolic rate is lowered;

Neurological disorders, especially cerebrovascular accident, which may be responsible not only for the initial fall causing exposure but, owing to the paralysis, also for limiting the heat generated by muscular activity;

Conditions associated with immobility – for example, stupor or coma from various causes, parkinsonism, paraplegia, and chronic arthritis. These patients are often confined to bed, and the lack of muscular activity leads to inadequate heat production;

Mental impairment and confusional states – if such patients are not receiving sufficient supervision they may be unable to protect themselves from cold exposure;

Severe infections and circulatory disturbances – for example, bronchopneumonia, cardiac infarction, and pulmonary embolism;

Drugs acting on the nervous system can further impair physiological mechanisms, particularly the phenothiazines, sedatives, antidepressives, and alcohol.

Thus a variety of acute and chronic conditions may be responsible, and in most cases of accidental hypothermia in the elderly both exogenous and endogenous factors operate in varying proportions.

Clinical features

A description of the clinical features is given in the reports of a series of cases treated in hospital by Duguid *et al*[7] and by Rosin and Exton-Smith.[8]

Appearance – The intense peripheral vasoconstriction leads to pallor of the skin, and when cyanosis is also present the patient looks pallid grey. There is puffiness of the face, and this together with the slow cerebration and the husky voice may be thought to be due to myxoedema.

Nervous system – As the body temperature falls below 32 °C clouding of consciousness, progressive confusion, and drowsiness develop. The patient's responses are slow and the reflexes are sluggish. Shivering is absent, and below about 30 °C it is replaced by a muscular hypertonus. This may lead to neck stiffness simulating meningism and to rigidity of the limbs. An involuntary flapping tremor in the arms and legs has been observed in some cases.[8]

Respiratory system – The respirations are slow and shallow. An appreciable fall in arterial oxygen saturation may occur as the result of this hypopnoea; the effect of anoxia on the tissue metabolism is one of the factors determining prognosis. Bronchopneumonia is nearly always present but it may not be detected owing to the absence of the usual clinical signs.

Cardiovascular system – In response to cold the heart rate slows due to sinus bradycardia or to slow atrial fibrillation. In the early stages the blood pressure is maintained, but a fall in blood pressure in spite of the intense peripheral vasoconstriction is a bad prognostic sign. The electrocardiogram often shows some degree of heart block with lengthening of the PR interval and delay in intraventricular conduction. A pathognomonic sign is the appearance of a J wave with characteristic deflection at the junction of the QRS and ST segments. These waves, which are usually best seen in V4, occur only in about a third of cases.

Alimentary system – Postmortem examination often shows acute pancreatitis, but the clinical diagnosis is rarely made. The clouding of consciousness and the muscular rigidity of the abdominal wall due to hypothermia obscure the usual signs, but pancreatitis should be suspected if the patient is seen to wince when firm pressure is applied to the epigastrium. The serum amylase activity is raised in most severe cases of hypothermia.

Management

A rapid restoration of normal temperature could ideally be expected to be the best method of treatment since it should avoid the complications resulting from prolonged hypothermia. In practice, however, it is a hazardous procedure in the elderly and frequently leads to circulatory collapse and an "after drop" in the

Management of accidental hypothermia

Mild hypothermia (deep body temperature 32–35 °C)
- (i) Room temperature of cubicle 25–30 °C; deep body temperature allowed to rise at about 0.5 °C/h.
- (ii) Barrier nursing. Administration of broad spectrum antibiotic.
- (iii) Controlled oxygen administration by means of a Venturi mask.
- (iv) Pulse and blood pressure monitoring; if there is a fall in the blood pressure during the treatment the patient is cooled again temporarily by lowering the room temperature.
- (v) Active measures for the prevention of pressure sores – for example, large cell ripple mattress.

Moderate to severe hypothermia (deep body temperature below 32 °C).
Additional measures to above requiring treatment in an intensive care unit
- (i) Institution of positive pressure ventilation to correct hypoxia and to re-expand collapsed alveoli.
- (ii) Insertion of central venous catheter for measurement of pressure and administration of warm fluids.
- (iii) The correction of dehydration and electrolyte disturbances.
- (iv) Loading dose of intravenous prophylactic antibiotic – for example, ampicillin or cloxacillin.
- (v) Monitoring of deep body temperature either continuously – for example, thermister in external auditory meatus or half hourly (rectal thermometer).
- (vi) ECG monitoring for cardiac arrhythmias.

---

core temperature which may precipitate cardiac arrhythmias. Normally for mild hypothermia (32–35 °C) it is not necessary to undertake active rewarming; the lightly covered patient should be nursed in a cubicle at an ambient temperature of 25–30 °C, and the body temperature should be allowed to come up very slowly (at about 0.5 °C per hour). According to the severity of the hypothermia one of the two therapeutic regimens summarised in the table should be instituted.

For some years now Ledingham[9] has adopted a more aggressive approach to the treatment of accidental hypothermia in the elderly – namely, actively rewarming, the institution of intermittent positive pressure ventilation, and the management of the patient in an intensive care unit. The effect of this regimen has been to eliminate deaths directly attributable to hypothermia, and by decreasing duration of recovery it has reduced the number of deaths indirectly attributable to this cause as well.

Preventive measures

Recognition of old people at risk

Doctors and community nurses should pay particular attention to old people living in cold accommodation even though they say they do not feel the cold. The regular recording of deep body temperature either by means of a low reading rectal thermometer or by the Uritemp technique, especially in those whose activities are restricted by chronic illness or disability, would be valuable. Social workers can detect many unmet needs in isolated old people and they should be aware of the circumstances that lead to accidental hypothermia.

Heating

As far as possible, elderly people should be encouraged to install in their homes safe means of heating – for example, electric convector heaters and night storage heaters. The heating of the bedroom is just as important as that of the sitting room. In severe weather when it may be impossible to keep more than one room warm it is preferable to have adequate heat in the living room and to make up the bed in it. Since many old people in receipt of supplementary benefits are not receiving an extra fuel allowance (largely because they do not know about it) wider publicity needs to be given to the availability of extra heating allowance (see Department of Health and Social Security[10]).

Clothing and blankets

Old people are sometimes found to be wearing unsuitable clothing, such as several felted woollen garments. For maximum comfort and warmth they should be advised that clothing needs to be light, closely woven, and not restricting. Similar comments also apply to bed clothes. Since many elderly people develop hypothermia at night the protection against exposure to cold while they are in bed is important. Although there may be some resistance to the use of a new appliance, an electric overblanket is very helpful. The conventional electric underblanket should not be used because of hazards in incontinent patients.

Nutrition

Many of the factors that make a person at risk of developing hypothermia also lead to malnutrition, so the two conditions are sometimes found together. The cost of extra fuel in winter may leave much less money to be spent on food. Many pensioners live on the borderline of malnutrition, and inadequate nutrition may occur just at the time when the energy needs of the body are greatest. It should be remembered, however, that it is not necessarily the thin, seemingly undernourished old people who are predisposed to hypothermia since they are more likely to be active; it can occur in the obese inactive old person. In spite of the feeling of warmth that alcohol gives, old people should be warned that it increases heat loss from the body and is conducive to hypothermia. In winter there is a need for the general practitioner and health visitor to pay particular attention to the adequacy and nutrient content of the diet of old people.

Conclusion

For the diagnosis of accidental hypothermia the deep body temperature must be measured either by means of a rectal thermometer or by the Uritemp technique. The much wider use of low reading thermometers by doctors and the community nursing services is essential, and there must be much greater awareness of the vulnerable groups in the elderly population. The early detection of accidental hypothermia in old people living at home and treatment before profound hypothermia has developed would seem to be the best means of reducing mortality.

1   Anonymous. Accidental hypothermia in the elderly. *Br Med J* 1964; ii: 1255.
2   Fox RH, Woodward PM, Exton-Smith AN, Green MF, Donnison DV, Wicks MH. Body temperatures in the elderly: a national study of physiological, social and environmental conditions. *Br Med J* 1973; i: 200–6.
3   Royal College of Physicians of London. *Report of committee on accidental hypothermia*. London: Royal College of Physicians, 1966.
4   Collins KJ, Doré C, Exton-Smith AN, Fox RH, MacDonald IC, Woodward PM. Accidental hypothermia and impaired temperature homoeostasis in the elderly. *Br Med J* 1977; i: 353–6.
5   Collins KJ, Easton JC, Exton-Smith AN. Shivering thermogenesis and vasomotor responses with convective cooling in the elderly. *J Physiol (Lond)* 1981; 20:76.
6   Collins KJ, Exton-Smith AN, Doré C. Urban hypothermia: preferred temperature and thermal perception in old age. *Br Med J* 1981; 282: 175–7.
7   Duguid H, Simpson RG, Stowers JM. Accidental hypothermia. *Lancet* 1961; ii: 1213–19.
8   Rosin A, Exton-Smith AN. Clinical features of accidental hypothermia with observations on thyroid function. *Br Med J* 1964; i: 16–9.
9   Ledingham IM. The clinical management of elderly hypothermic patients. In: Pozos RS, Wittmers LE, eds. *The nature and treatment of hypothermia*. London: Croom Helm, 1983.
10 Department of Health and Social Security. *Keeping warm in winter*. London: HMSO, 1972.

Cardiovascular disease in the old

J WEDGWOOD

In many cases cardiovascular disease in the old is similar to the disease in the young and middle aged except that its pathology is weighted towards conditions such as ischaemic heart disease rather than congenital or rheumatic heart disease. This point, though perhaps obvious, needs to be made to emphasise that most forms of heart disease in the young that do not cause early death may be found in old age.

In other cases, particularly those presenting to the geriatric physician and in patients over 75 or 80 years, the aetiology, symptoms, course, and response to treatment are all considerably modified and need separate consideration. This chapter is concerned with this group of patients and will deal with the commoner conditions in which the differences are most appreciable and which present particular problems to the general practitioner. Congestive heart failure is a common condition covering most aspects of heart disease, and so this chapter will be limited to a discussion of this condition.

The most outstanding feature of congestive heart failure is the ease with which elderly patients develop it and the relatively good response to treatment.[1] Congestive failure may develop in patients with less clinical evidence of heart disease than would be expected in younger patients. Though there is usually evidence of myocardial or valvular heart disease, precipitating factors are particularly important and need to be recognised before the condition can be adequately treated.

Precipitating factors

Chest infection is a particularly important factor to bear in mind. Signs of bronchopneumonia may be difficult to detect, and relatively slight infection is often sufficient to precipitate failure. The combination of chest infection and heart failure in which it is

Lead

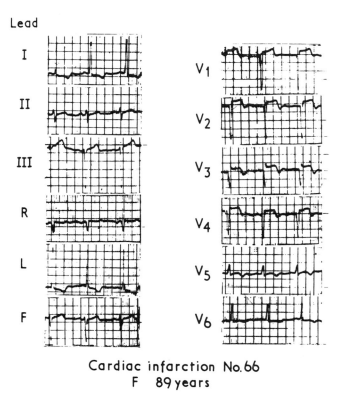

Cardiac infarction No.66
F   89 years

FIG 1 *Acute anterior infarction in 89 year old woman without symptoms.* (By kind permission of the publisher[8])

difficult to decide the relative contribution of pulmonary and cardiac factors is common.

Atrial fibrillation is common in the elderly and may be paroxysmal. When the ventricular rate is rapid it is a common cause of failure. A more serious arrhythmia is atrial flutter or atrial tachycardia with atrioventricular block. This condition is difficult to detect clinically except by inspection of the venous pulse. When atrioventricular block is present with a 2:1 ventricular response the ventricular rate may be relatively slow and regular. It is particularly likely to occur in a patient who is being treated with digitalis for atrial fibrillation. It is a serious complication of digitalis toxicity, easily missed, and likely to be fatal.[2]

Heart block – When the ventricular rate is slow heart block may be a cause of congestive failure; this responds to measures which increase the ventricular rate. Stokes Adams attacks are the more

97

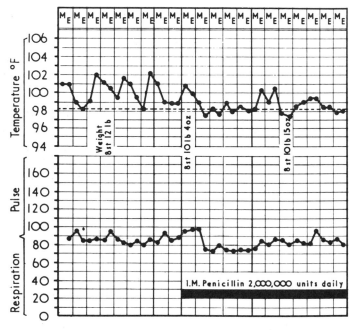

FIG 2 *Unexpected fever in a 69 year old woman with infective endocarditis.*

dramatic effects of heart block, but congestive failure, chronic ill health, and confusional states may also be features of the slow ventricular rate. Artificial pacemaking is of value in these patients, and age should not prevent its use.

The "sick sinus" syndrome is not strictly relevant to congestive failure but deserves mention because of the possibility that an attack of paroxysmal supraventricular tachycardia may be a manifestation of this syndrome. If this be the case appropriate medication may be followed by a disproportionately severe bradycardia. Awareness of this possibility is necessary. Diagnosis must rest on 24 hour electrocardiographic monitoring. The treatment is not easy and may best be dealt with by a pacemaker combined with an anti-arrhythmic drug.

Cardiac infarction – Silent cardiac infarction is common in the old or may present with minor symptoms of confusion, weakness, or syncope, without chest pain (fig 1).[3] It may also present with congestive failure and should be suspected in patients who develop failure without obvious cause. Clinical support for this diagnosis may be obtained from the sudden development of a triple rhythm, which is often most easily heard over the lower sternum or xiphoid process in the old when auscultation is difficult.[4]

Infective endocarditis is common in old age, and the diagnosis is often missed.[5-7] The insidious onset in the old may be associated with "unexplained" congestive failure. It should be suspected in patients with congestive heart failure, a heart murmur, and disproportionate ill health, particularly if fever is present (fig 2).

Other conditions which precipitate failure and may easily be missed are anaemia, thyrotoxicosis, myxoedema, and salt retention due to treatment with steroids or with stilboestrol for carcinoma of the prostate. Pulmonary embolism is a fairly frequent cause of failure. Deep vein thrombosis is common and easily missed. Recurrent pulmonary embolism as a cause of failure may be difficult to diagnose.

Underlying factors

In most elderly patients myocardial disease is the underlying cause of failure. In about a quarter of the cases evidence of previous cardiac infarction or the presence of hypertension supports a diagnosis of ischaemic heart disease (table).[8] The remaining cases are usually considered to have ischaemic heart disease on rather less evidence. The precision of this diagnosis may be questioned but it remains a useful term and preferable to the obsolete "senile myocardial degeneration" which it replaced.

The postmortem finding of brown atrophy of the myocardium is not related to the presence of failure. The finding of amyloid

Heart disease on discharge or death in patients aged 80 years and over

	Men	Women	Total (No)	Total (%)
Ischaemic heart disease without infarction	75	69	144	73
Ischaemic heart disease with infarction	19	20	39	20
Ischaemic heart disease with hypertension	0	6	6	3
Valvular heart disease	3	3	6	3
Cor pulmonale	2	1	3	1
Totals	99	99	198	100

By kind permission of the publishers.[8]

deposits in the heart muscle of elderly patients dying of congestive failure has received much attention.[9,10] Its incidence varies considerably in published series but is particularly high in those over 90. Its clinical significance is debatable.

Valvular and congenital heart disease, cor pulmonale

Nearly all forms of congenital heart disease, except those associated with an early mortality, and of rheumatic and syphilitic heart disease have been found in old age (figs 3 and 4).[8] Cor pulmonale occurs in elderly patients but is rare in the type of patient discussed here; though combinations of failure, chest infection, and emphysema, in which the aetiology is mixed, are common. Probably patients with congenital lesions or valvular heart disease acquired in earlier adult life who survive to these late ages do not develop failure until a myocardial factors is introduced.

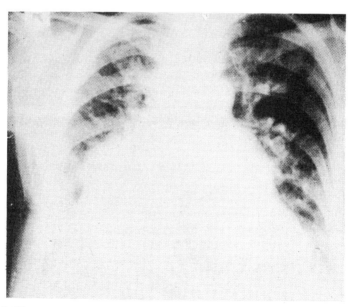

FIG 3 *Chest x ray film from 79 year old woman with a ventricular septal defect confirmed at necropsy.* (By kind permission of the publishers of *Practitioner* and of Dr K M MacKenzie[11])

Some forms of valvular heart disease, particularly mitral incompetence, may develop in old age as a result of cardiac infarction, ischaemic heart disease, calcification, or degenerative changes.

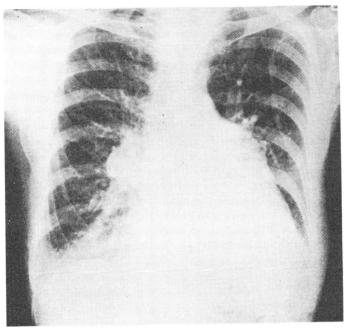

FIG 4 *Chest x ray film from 75 year old woman with an atrial septal defect.*

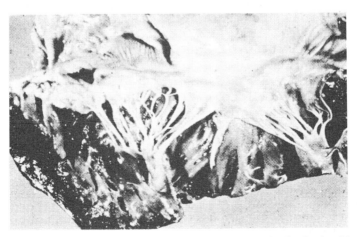

FIG 5 *Necropsy specimen showing degenerative changes in the mitral valve in a 90 year old woman with mitral incompetence and intractable failure.* (By courtesy of Dr G Farrer-Brown, Bland-Sutton Institute, The Middlesex Hospital Medical School)

101

Calcification of the mitral valve ring (fig 5), mitral valve prolapse, and changes in the chordae tendineae or papillary muscles may all cause mitral incompetence.

An important problem also is severe aortic stenosis due to calcification of the aortic valve. The clinical signs of aortic stenosis may be difficult to interpret in these cases, and the condition is easily missed.

The difficulty of auscultation and the fact that investigation is often not practical mean that our power of diagnosis in these cases is restricted. The situation has been improved by echocardiography. The selection of patients for this non-invasive procedure, from the large number of elderly people with systolic murmurs, is not easy; but it should be considered if the patient is fit for cardiac surgery and an operable lesion is suspected. Systolic murmurs are difficult to assess, they may vary in length with the cardiac output, originate from more than one valve, or originate in an extracardiac arterial bruit in the abdomen or neck.

It is often difficult to estimate the haemodynamic significance of a suspected valvular lesion, but the importance of mitral incompetence or aortic stenosis as a cause of failure is easy to underestimate. The presence of a heart murmur should also be taken seriously because of the risk of infective endocarditis.

Hypertension

Hypertensive heart disease is rare in the type of patient discussed here, though some degree of hypertension with ischaemic heart disease is common. The indication for using hypotensive drugs in those over 75, either for the relief of failure or on general principles, is infrequent. These drugs should hardly ever be used because of the risks of reducing the cerebral blood flow.

Diagnosis

It is necessary to emphasise the importance of accurate diagnosis in congestive failure. The term is often used imprecisely to explain weakness, shortness of breath, or oedema of the ankles – for which there are many causes other than heart failure. Correct diagnosis is difficult but important since an incorrect diagnosis of heart failure may greatly restrict the patient's rehabilitation and independence.

The diagnosis of congestive heart failure rests on careful examination of the venous pulse in the internal jugular vein. This is difficult in the old because of senile kyphosis and the problem of positioning the patient. Arterial abnormalities in the neck may cause unusual pulsations or on the left side cause pressure effects that mimic a raised venous pressure.[12,13] Inspection should therefore be made of the righthand side of the neck, and, if there is difficulty in distinguishing an arterial from a venous pulse, pressure over the liver will raise an abnormal venous pulse and over the lower part of the neck obliterate it.

Other signs of heart failure in the elderly tend to have equivocal significance. Rales at the lung bases can be found in many elderly patients who have been in bed.[14] The liver edge may be palpable owing to a low diaphragm or deformed rib cage. Oedema of the legs is common in the elderly without heart failure, though a sacral pad of oedema is perhaps more significant.

These difficulties emphasise the need for negative diagnosis. If the heart is not enlarged, there are no abnormal heart sounds, and the electrocardiogram is normal heart failure is unlikely to be present. Palpation of the apex beat, auscultation, a chest x ray film, and an electrocardiogram may be helpful in a negative way.

Treatment

The importance of precipitating factors in heart failure in the old has been mentioned, and their recognition and treatment are of great importance. The diagnosis and treatment of concomitant chest infection with an appropriate antibiotic need particular emphasis. Signs in the chest may be minimal, and it is often justifiable to give an antibiotic on the suspicion that infection may be present if the response to treatment has otherwise been poor.

Diuretics

In the absence of atrial fibrillation diuretics and the treatment of the precipitating cause are usually all that is needed. Digitalis should be kept in reserve unless atrial fibrillation is present. The choice and method of giving diuretics must take into account the problem of incontinence and, in men, retention of urine if there is some prostatic obstruction. Elderly people may be weakened by the effort required to deal with a massive diuresis and do not stand up well to rapid changes in fluid and electrolyte balance. In most cases there is no need for the vigorous use of diuretics or for the more complex potent diuretics required in younger patients with severe or resistant failure.

The method and frequency of administration need thought. Elderly patients may not take tablets regularly or may spit them out after the nurse has left; in them the parenteral route may be better than the oral. After the acute phase is over diuretics may not need to be given daily. In maintenance therapy the diuretic can be given intermittently on the most convenient days. The patient should be regularly assessed and maintenance diuretics stopped as soon as possible. Diuretics tend to be continued after the problem of congestive failure has receded, from habit and because of the difficulty in deciding that heart failure has stopped in the presence of factors such as leg oedema. If diuretics are given in small doses, intermittently, and for short periods their complications such as potassium deficiency, gout, and the provocation of diabetes, are less likely to occur and the patient's regimen is more easily managed.

Many of the above principles may seem obvious but are often neglected and more attention given to the nature of the diuretic itself. The choice of diuretic is of less importance except that the more potent and complex diuretic programmes are rarely needed. In the more serious or acute conditions a loop diuretic such as frusemide has the advantage of powerful action, flexibility of dosage, and oral or parenteral administration. Given by mouth it acts within one hour and lasts for about eight hours. Its disadvantage is that it may be too effective – a problem that may be diminished by giving it in the smallest possible dose.

In less serious states and for maintenance the thiazides are satisfactory. They act more slowly (within four hours) and last longer (for about 12 hours). Their prolonged action may be a handicap.

The aldosterone antagonists should only be considered when failure is difficult to treat or there are problems of induced hypokalaemia. They are powerful drugs and require good patient compliance, with careful clinical and electrolyte monitoring. If these conditions cannot be implemented their use is difficult.

Potassium supplements

Potassium deficiency may be troublesome in the old and aggravate digitalis toxicity. Its occurrence is reduced if the general principles outlined are adhered to, but some form of potassium supplement is usually needed if the thiazides or frusemide are given. Such supplements do not obviate the need for regular assessment of patients on long term diuretics. Though extra tablets are a nuisance for elderly patients, potassium supplements may be more easily controlled if given separately. The thiazide diuretics with slow release potassium offer the advantages of ease of administration but the disadvantage of a relatively small dose of potassium.

The danger of hypokalaemia has to be balanced against the likelihood of its occurrence (the patient's size, diet, and dose of diuretics), and against the risk of inducing hyperkalaemia. Regular electrolyte estimations are not easy in disabled patients living at home. The most important aspect of diuretic therapy is to give diuretics only when necessary, to stop diuretics as soon as possible, and to watch the patient's general condition. It should always be borne in mind that deterioration in a patient, however well the congestive failure may be responding to treatment, may be a result of diuretics, electrolyte disturbance, or digitalis.

Digitalis

Digitalisation is a considerable problem in elderly patients: digitalis intoxication is easily produced with small doses of the drug.[15] Mental confusion[16] is often the first indication of overdosage, or the patient may look or feel ill. Nausea and vomiting may occur later. These symptoms are insidious and easily missed. The illness produced by digitalis in elderly patients has a most deleterious effect on their recovery, apart from the danger of atrial or ventricular

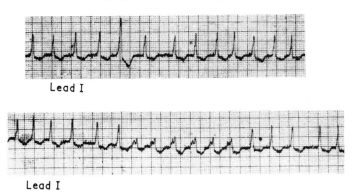

FIG 6 *Ectopic arrhythmia due to digitalis. ECG lead II. Woman aged 90 years* (By kind permission of the publishers of *Modern Medicine.*)

arrhythmias – which are common (fig 6), more difficult to treat in the elderly than in the young, and often fatal. Digitalis needs to be given cautiously and the individual's response to it assessed by giving low doses in the first instance. Digoxin has the advantage of relatively quick action and excretion. Digoxin 0.25 mg three times a day is a large dose in old age, and 0.25 mg once or twice a day is often sufficient for the initial period. The maintenance dosage needs to be much smaller – 0.125 mg or 0.0625 mg daily. Frequent observation of the patient is needed in the early stages of treatment for early symptoms or signs, particularly arrhythmias, of digitalis overdose. These should be taken seriously and the drug stopped at once if they occur. The danger of a large diuresis, or of potassium deficiency, aggravating the effects of digitalis should be borne in mind. Patients on long term digitalis should be reviewed regularly, and unless there is good reason for continuing to give the drug it should be stopped.

Vasodilators: preload and afterload reduction

The value of these measures in the elderly has to be established. They may involve complex drug regimens which produce problems of patient compliance, monitoring, and side effects. They should probably be reserved at present for use in special circumstances but may need to be considered if other methods fail.[17]

In general it cannot be overemphasised that the usual problem in an elderly patient with heart failure, who does not appear to be responding to treatment, is a simple one; the diagnosis is wrong or a simple cause, such as an occult chest infection, has been missed. This possibility should always be carefully considered before embarking on complex alterations of treatment.

Conclusion

The symptomatology and course of cardiovascular disease is modified by age, and there are several forms of heart disease specific to old age. Congestive failure is a common and often complex problem. With accurate diagnosis and careful treatment the prognosis is relatively good. The paradox of cardiovascular disease in the old is that, though heart disease is common in patients who survive to advanced old age, they are a selected group, a biological élite, whose general health and hearts might be expected to be unusually good.

I thank Dr G Farrer-Brown for permission to publish fig 5.

[1] Bedford PD, Caird FI. Congestive heart failure in the elderly. *Q J Med* 1956; **25**: 407–26.
[2] Lown B, Levine SA. *Current concepts in digitalis therapy*. London: Churchill, 1955.
[3] Pathy MS. Clinical presentation of myocardial infarction in the elderly. *Br Heart J* 1967; **29**; 190–9.
[4] Evans WE. Triple heart rhythm. *Br Heart J* 1943; **5**: 205–28.
[5] Lerner PI, Weinstein L. Infective endocarditis in the antibiotic era. *N Engl J Med* 1966; **274**: 199–206, 259–66, 388–93.
[6] Wedgwood J. Early diagnosis of subacute bacterial endocarditis. *Lancet* 1955; ii: 1058–63.
[7] Wedgwood J. In: Caird FI, Dall JLC, Kennedy RD, eds. *Cardiology in old age*. New York and London: Plenum Press, 1976: 230.
[8] Wedgwood J. Clinical aspects of ischaemic heart disease in old age. In: Agate JN, ed. *Medicine in old age*. London: Pitman Medical, 1966: 216–26.

9 McKeown F. Heart disease in old age. *J Clin Pathol* 1963; **16**: 532–7.
10 Pomerance A. Senile cardiac amyloidosis. *Br Heart J* 1965; **27**: 711–8.
11 Wedgwood J. Cardiovascular disease in the elderly. *Practitioner* 1968; **200**: 778–85.
12 Smith KS. The kinked innominate vein. *Br Heart J* 1960; **22**: 110–6.
13 Sleight P. Unilateral elevation of the internal jugular pulse. *Br Heart J* 1962; **24**: 726–30.
14 Wood P. *Diseases of the heart and circulation.* 2nd ed. London: Eyre and Spottiswoode, 1956.
15 Wedgwood J. Therapeutic topics. The use and abuse of digitalis. *Modern Geriatrics* 1970; **1**; 40–4.
16 Duroziez P. *Gazette Hebdomadaire de Médecine et de Chirurgie* 1874; **2**: 780.
17 Hamer J. In: Martin A, Camn AJ, eds. *Heart disease in the elderly.* Chichester: John Wiley and Sons, 1984: 187–203.

Urinary tract diseases in the elderly

B MOORE-SMITH

Four aspects of urinary tract disease are discussed – uraemia, prostatic disease, urinary tract infection, and incontinence – and attention is drawn to some features of these conditions of particular importance in the elderly.

Uraemia

The finding of a moderately raised blood urea concentration (8–12 mmol/l (48–72 mg/100 ml)) in elderly patients is so common that it is often regarded as normal – in the sense that it requires no immediate correction and is not accompanied by identifiable symptoms. As a chance finding it suggests an aging kidney with progressive nephron depletion, providing a warning that the stability of the patient's internal environment may be threatened and carrying therapeutic implications for the many drugs excreted through, or potentially toxic to, the kidney.

The causes of uraemia may be divided into three – prerenal, renal, and postrenal – but all of these, of course, may be superimposed on existing nephron loss in an aging kidney.

Prerenal uraemia

Prerenal uraemia is due to inadequate glomerular filtration caused usually by such factors as haemorrhage, loss of extracellular fluid, or severely impaired cardiac output. In the elderly some degree of dehydration, based on inadequate intake, perhaps through fear of later incontinence, is common. Any further factor such as diarrhoea and vomiting, a silent myocardial infarction, or unmonitored diuretic therapy may produce an acute uraemic state, with confusion often as its leading symptom. The blood urea concentration may be as high as 33–42 mmol/l (198–253 mg/100 ml) and will rapidly fall with adequate rehydration. A distinguishing feature in such cases is the maintenance of a normal or only moderately reduced plasma bicarbonate concentration.

Renal uraemia

Any diffuse renal disease may be present in the elderly, but probably the most common is chronic pyelonephritis. Diabetic nephropathy is less common, though diabetes is a common condition. The various forms of glomerulonephritis have their incidence chiefly earlier in life, and hypertensive renal disease likewise is relatively uncommon.

Postrenal uraemia

The key to postrenal uraemia is obstruction to the flow of urine anywhere in the urinary passages. In both sexes chronic retention of urine based on faecal impaction is by no means uncommon and reinforces the necessity for routine rectal examination in the elderly. In men the commonest cause is prostatic enlargement, and as many as 30% of men aged 80 or over have appreciable enlargement and often impaired flow.[1] In women obstruction is less common but the presence of a cystocele may impair flow, and, particularly with complete procidentia, severe back pressure effects may result with the development of silent hydronephrosis. In these circumstances sudden death from acute renal failure over a matter of days may occur following a trivial alteration in renal perfusion.

Management

Management of acute renal failure by purely medical means is the same as in younger age groups and will not be discussed. The management of chronic uraemia depends primarily on the cause. The most immediately remediable causes, also the commonest, lie in the prerenal group, and here the recognition of states of dehydration is important while treatment with oral fluids is straightforward provided it is adequately supervised. If there is any question of appreciable gastrointestinal tract loss appropriate replacement of electrolyte deficiencies is essential. A full assessment of the cardiovascular system, including an electrocardiogram, is necessary in any case of unexplained uraemia.

In postrenal causes of uraemia relief of the cause of the obstruction is a priority and age per se is no contraindication to surgery. The criterion for operation is the total clinical condition of the patient.

Provided underlying renal function is preserved, relief of prerenal and postrenal factors will eliminate uraemia; in chronic renal failure, however, relief of the cause may well be impossible, and treatment then becomes a matter of compensation for the renal defect so far as is possible. Age over 60 has been shown to be a major determinant of success for both renal dialysis and transplantation. The risk of mortality with age is less in patients on dialysis (79 % survival at one year compared with 65 % for transplantation).[2] Concomitant disease and disability become commoner with increasing age, and among the developed countries, in the United Kingdom especially, there is also the question of the rationing of resources. In the management of chronic renal failure in the elderly it is especially important to ensure that the treatment is not worse than the disease and that the measures are simple and therefore more likely to be carried out. The following are some points to observe.

Fluid intake – Urea excretion is proportional to urine flow, and with low urinary output a slowly increasing "head" of urea and other metabolites builds up in the plasma. This may be reduced by increasing the volume of urine passed and therefore the solute load excreted, even when the number of residual functioning nephrons is very severely reduced. It may, however, be difficult to persuade the elderly of the need to drink large quantities of fluid, and resistance to advice may be great, especially if there is a pre-existing degree of incontinence or if lavatory facilities are inadequate. Even a moderate increase in urine flow is beneficial over a period of time. The help of relatives is invaluable in treating the patient outside hospital.

Ionic balance – Sodium depletion may occur because of reduced sodium conservation and can cause further deterioration of renal function, particularly during incidental illness. Potassium retention is well known with its dangers to the myocardium, and foods of high potassium content should be avoided as a general rule. A degree of acidosis is common but is usually well tolerated.

Protein – The elderly frequently eat a relatively high carbohydrate, low protein diet, and dietary control is not a major problem. Older people do not tolerate change, and extreme dietary restrictions are not likely to be observed.

Anaemia – Anaemia is invariable, usually well tolerated, and is unresponsive to haematinics. Transfusion is only temporarily effective, hazardous, and best avoided.

Drugs – All drugs are potentially toxic, and the aging nephron-depleted kidney is prone to drug induced damage, especially by analgesics containing phenacetin, salicylate, and paracetamol. It also produces higher serum concentrations of drugs whose excretion is primarily renal and so greater renal and extra renal toxicity. In this latter instance aminoglycoside and cephalosporin antibiotics should be used with care and nalidixic acid, nitrofurantoin, and tetracyclines, except doxycycline and minocycline, should be avoided. Many other drugs should be used with great caution in the elderly with aging kidneys, including such diverse examples as allopurinol, chlorpropamide, cimetidine, and thiazides. There are recent succinct reviews of the problems of drugs and the kidney available.[3,4]

Prostatic disease

The usual presentation of prostatic disease – increasing difficulty in micturition – may be masked in the elderly, and the initial symptoms may be haematuria or, as with younger patients, acute retention precipitated by diuretic therapy or anticholinergic drugs. Less widely recognised perhaps are dribbling incontinence due to retention with overflow and unrecognised acute retention causing a confusional state. A uraemic syndrome in a man always requires exclusion of prostatic obstruction as a cause. Treatment is essentially surgical, and the results are good in suitable patients at any age. The relative simplicity, in experienced hands, of transurethral resection carries lower morbidity and mortality than open operation.

Carcinoma of the prostate is the commonest neoplastic disease of elderly men, said to be present in 95 % of histologically examined prostates in those aged over 70.[5] Presentation may be through urinary symptoms but not uncommonly is due to metastatic disease. In particular, the diagnosis should be considered in previously fit men in their 80s and 90s who complain of nothing more than mild malaise or whose social behaviour deteriorates for no apparent reason over a short time. Bone pain, particularly in the lumbosacral spine or pelvis, is a relatively frequent metastatic presentation, but very widespread bony metastases may be asymptomatic. The plasma acid phosphatase activity is variable but is frequently raised, sometimes to very high activities, and with extensive bone involvement a raised alkaline phosphatase activity and sometimes a peripheral blood picture of leucoerythroblastic anaemia may be seen. Treatment by orchidectomy or with oestrogens in most instances is successful, and lengthy remissions are frequently seen.

Urinary tract infection

The spontaneous rate of urinary tract infection in women seen in domiciliary practice is said to be around 2 %, but surveys of the elderly at home have found rates of around 20 % in Britain,[6,7] and in hospital rates as high as 67 % have been quoted[8]; in men spontaneous infection below the age of 70 is rare but its occurrence is said to be similar to that in women above this age. Possibly a prostatic antibacterial factor may account for this difference between the sexes at younger ages.[9] In elderly men collection of a reliable midstream urine specimen (MSU) is relatively straightforward; in elderly women, on the other hand, it is a task of some difficulty, and the average MSU is almost certainly not midstream and infrequently composed solely of urine. Thus urine specimens from elderly women submitted for bacteriological examination are often contaminated from various sources and this is reflected in the reported results of culture, before which the specimens may frequently be "incubated" at room temperature for several hours. This last difficulty is obviated by "dip slide" techniques, but the provenance of the specimen "dipped" still remains in some doubt. In hospital conditions MSUs in elderly women have been shown to have a 57 % false positive rate,[10] and, though suprapubic aspiration gives reliable specimens, it is technically unsuitable for routine use. Alexa bag specimens show a similar order of reliability and can be used to check "abnormal" MSUs.

The interpretation of the results of laboratory examination depends primarily on the quantitative bacterial count. Significant infection is associated only with bacterial counts above $100 \times 10^6/1$.[11] There must be only one organism, and in domiciliary practice this is likely to be *Escherichia coli* or *Proteus* spp in a pure culture. Two or more organisms reported as coexisting are due to contamination no matter how high the count. The presence or absence of pus cells is in general unhelpful, and microscopical haematuria is uncommon.[10]

Differentiation between upper and lower urinary tract infection in the elderly is difficult clinically. The classic clinical picture of acute pyelonephritis is uncommon, and chronic pyelonephritis, though common (6 % in one survey[12]) as a postmortem finding, is seldom accompanied by local symptoms in life.[13-16] In contrast to much current belief and teaching, use of a simple localisation technique has recently shown that 55 % of urinary tract infections in elderly women, admitted acutely to a geriatric unit, affect the kidneys.[17]

Significant bacteriuria is often asymptomatic in the elderly. It is usually assumed that it should be treated because of the deleterious effects of urinary infection on renal function, which is already likely to be compromised, as well as the known high incidence of pyelonephritis. There is, however, no good evidence that this view is correct, and clinically many elderly catheterised patients tolerate their inevitable urinary infections well especially if fluids are greatly encouraged.

Treatment

Dilution of antibiotic concentration by a high fluid intake during treatment is far outweighed by the decreased reproduction rate of *E coli* in diluted urine and the washout effect of the high urine flow on the bacterial numbers. The vast majority of *E coli* found in domiciliary practice are still sensitive to sulphonamides which are safe and effective. Otherwise, antibiotic treatment should follow the sensitivities found on culture and with appropriate manipulation of the urinary pH to match the organism concerned and the antibiotic chosen.

The length of treatment for a straightforward urinary infection is customarily one week, although ultra-short courses are growing in popularity.[18] Acute pyelonephritis is usually treated for two weeks. In chronic pyelonephritis recommendations for length of treatment vary from six weeks to six months, using rotating antibiotics, but there is little further evidence of their efficacy or necessity. A short (two week) initial course with careful follow up is probably preferable.

Relapse or reinfection is as common as in younger age groups; if it persists investigation is required, as treatment will be without lasting benefit until the cause is eliminated. By the same token a urinary infection should always be checked after treatment to confirm relief and, if pyelonephritis is suspected, at monthly intervals for six months.

Incontinence

When the intravesical pressure exceeds the urethral resistance voiding normally occurs; voiding becomes incontinence when it happens in an uncontrolled fashion. In the elderly lack of adequate higher cerebral control is often an important cause, though the local mechanisms remain intact. This is seen transiently in early strokes, acute confusional episodes and states of altered consciousness, and epilepsy. It may also be seen in some frontal lobe lesions and particularly in established dementia.

Despite normal higher cerebral control environmental factors may be vitally important as a source of apparent incontinence when access to the lavatory is restricted or it is too far away, or toilet rounds are inflexible, or attendants fail to realise that the matter is urgent. Being bedfast or chairfast are powerful overriding factors. Rarely with normal high control and intact bladder mechanisms psychological factors may underlie apparent incontinence as a facet of a "call for help."

Local causes affecting the bladder mechanisms may overstimulate the detrusor by irritating it, as in acute cystitis, bladder stone, or neoplasm. All these cause urgency, and incontinence if help is not at hand. How far urinary infection on its own is responsible for incontinence is less certain. After many months of contracting against prostatic obstruction the detrusor may dilate, become unable to expel the last part of the urine, and finally become an inert and grossly distended bag stretching the bladder neck and causing continuous dribbling incontinence. Stress incontinence in women is fairly common in the elderly and depends on the altered anatomical relationship between the bladder neck and urethra, on the one hand, and the pelvic floor, on the other. Urethral resistance is sometimes diminished by invasion by prostatic carcinoma resulting in dribbling incontinence; otherwise, urethral malfunction is almost unknown as a cause of incontinence.

Interference with the nerve supply to the bladder will also interfere with the balance between the detrusor and the urethra plus the external sphincter. Thus incontinence may result from a wide variety of causes, from cerebral lesions to peripheral neuropathy. In multiple sclerosis, for instance, there is frequently a progression from detrusor overactivity early, with incontinence, to increased outflow resistance later, with retention.

Treatment

Local causes require local treatment and must always be sought before accepting incontinence as being due to loss of higher control. The transient causes may be allowed to resolve as the underlying condition improves, while environmental factors in particular should be amenable to alteration and explanation. The importance of getting the patient out of bed with its connotations of helpless dependence cannot be overemphasised. Also of vital importance are the avoidance of unnecessary hypnotics and the initiation of regular toiletting and habit training, which can often greatly improve incontinence of so called cerebral origin. Surgical help should always be sought in appropriate circumstances.

In some instances, despite correction of all remediable abnormalities, the patient is left with intractable incontinence. In women, especially if confused, it is impossible to fit an adequate external appliance, though some devices are suitable for the mentally alert and well motivated. A catheter is therefore the only practical solution and if of small size, with a small bag and adequately cared for, success for a period of years can be obtained with infection rarely a major problem. In men long term catheterisation can cause troublesome periurethral problems, but in practice the relief to all concerned outweighs these dangers, and a successful catheter life can be led for many months or even years. Before inserting a catheter, however, consideration should be given to the wide variety of incontinence appliances available. If fitted carefully these may be of considerable help, especially when the patient is out of bed. Nearly all appliances suffer from reflux problems in bed, and considerable cooperation by the patient is needed for success. Electronic implants for increasing outflow resistance may help in selected patients of both sexes and are under continuing development.

1 Agate JN. *The practice of geriatrics.* 2nd ed. London: William Heinemann Medical Books, 1970: 428.
2 Matthew TH. An integrated approach to terminal renal failure. *Medicine International* 1982; 1, 23: 1090–1.
3 Cove-Smith R. Drugs and the kidney. *Medicine International* 1982; 1, 24: 1124–38.
4 Adu D. Drug induced renal diseases. *Prescribers Journal* 1984; 24, 3: 46–51.
5 Agate JN. *The practice of geriatrics.* 2nd ed. London: William Heinemann Medical Books, 1970: 429.
6 Brocklehurst JC, Dulane JB, Griffiths L, Fry J. The prevalence and symptomatology of urinary infection in an aged population. *Gerontologia Clinica* 1968; 10: 242–53.
7 Akthar HR, Andrew GR, Caird F, Fallow RJ. Urinary tract infection in the elderly; a population study. *Age Ageing* 1972; 1: 48–54.
8 McMillan J, Linton AL. Urinary tract infection in old age. *Gerontologia Clinica* 1968; 10: 58–62.
9 Stamey TA, Fair WR, Timothy MM, Chung HK. Antibacterial nature of prostatic fluid. *Nature* 1968; 218: 444–7.
10 Moore-Smith B. Suprapubic aspiration in the diagnosis of urinary infection in the elderly. *Modern Geriatrics* 1971; 1: 124–9.
11 Kass EH. Asymptomatic infections in the urinary tract. *Transactions of the Association of American Physicians* 1956; 69: 56–64.
12 Kass EH. In: Quinn EL, Kass EH, eds. *Biology of pyelonephritis.* Little Brown: Boston, 1960: 399.
13 Mond NC, Percival A, Williams JD, Brumfitt W. Presentation, diagnosis and treatment of urinary tract infections in general practice. *Lancet* 1965; i: 514–9.
14 Fairley KF, Carson NE, Gutchm RC, *et al.* Site of infection in acute urinary tract infection in general practice. *Lancet* 1971; ii: 615–8.
15 Boutros P, Mourtada H, Ronald AR. Urinary infection localisation. *Am J Obstet Gynecol* 1972; 112: 379–81.
16 Smeets F, Gower PE. The site of infection in 133 patients with bacteriuria. *Clin Nephrol* 1973; 1: 290–6.
17 Suntharalingham M, Seth V, Moore-Smith B. Site of urinary tract infection in elderly women admitted to an acute geriatric assessment unit. *Age Ageing* 1983; 12: 317–22.
18 Bailey RR. Ed. *Single dose therapy of urinary tract infection.* Sydney: ADIS Health Science Press, 1983.

Problems of interpretation of laboratory findings in the old

F I CAIRD

Haematological, biochemical, and endocrine disorders are common in old age and are often eminently remediable, but assessment of their importance is often hampered by problems of interpretation of the laboratory data on which the diagnosis and management of such disorders usually rest. There are several reasons for these difficulties in interpretation. Simple lack of knowledge of well established normal values is common. Many normal values in the elderly are identical to those recognised for the young. If an abnormal value is mistakenly considered to be normal "for the patient's age," the opportunity for correct diagnosis and active treatment will be missed. Conversely, some normal values differ in the elderly from those taught for the young. If a value normal for the patient's age is considered abnormal the patient may be subjected to unnecessary and possibly even hazardous further investigations – or an incorrect diagnosis and so perhaps prognosis may result. In both instances reference ranges which take age (and so many patients) into account are rarely given, while the necessary information may be found only in journals which are not easily accessible, may not yet be in the textbooks, and in consequence is not commonly taught.

A further difficulty arises from the fact that some normal values are not yet certainly established for the elderly. One main reason for this is the high frequency of disease states in old age, which greatly affects results but to a variable extent. Those from hospital series and those from old people at home may differ considerably. A clear definition of the population used is vital. Other reasons for differences between published series are methodological, inappropriate statistics, and the variable but high use of drugs, which may affect a wide range of tests. There is often in addition a problem in assessing the significance of minor deviations from normality as shown by laboratory tests in old people and consequent difficulty in management of patients with such abnormalities.

This chapter attempts to review and discuss with respect to the elderly several commonly performed laboratory tests and the problems of interpretation which they present, both in relation to screening procedures and to the assessment of sick old people.

Haematological tests

Haemoglobin concentrations

The haemoglobin concentration does not change significantly with age,[1,2] and thus values considered to indicate anaemia should be identical in young and old. If a haemoglobin concentration of less than 12 g/dl is taken to define anaemia,[3] or at least as an indication for further investigation, a few elderly women will be found whose haemoglobin concentration lies between 11.5 and 11.9 g/dl yet who have no evident cause for anaemia[4] and several men will be overlooked whose haemoglobin concentration is above 12 g/dl yet who have a definite and diagnosable abnormality remediable by treatment. Nevertheless, 12 g/dl is probably the best single concentration for the definition of anaemia in old age.

The standard haematological indices (mean cell haemoglobin, mean corpuscular volume, etc) and the appearances of the blood film are unaffected by age. A low mean cell haemoglobin concentration and hypochromia should thus be taken to indicate iron deficiency, at least in the first instance, since this is much the commonest single cause of anaemia in old people at home,[4,5] though secondary hypochromic anaemia due to a wide range of causes is also very common in elderly hospital patients. A low serum ferritin concentration may help to discriminate.

Similarly anaemia, a high mean cell volume, and macrocytosis are evidence of the need to exclude a megaloblastic state due to deficiency of vitamin B_{12} or folate. A raised mean cell volume without anaemia is commonly due to a chronic high alcohol intake.[6] This is as true of the elderly as of the young.

Serum iron concentrations

The serum iron tends to fall with age,[2,7] so that concentrations as low as 5–6 μmol/l (28–34 μg/100 ml) may be found when iron stores are adequate, as shown by the presence of substantial amounts in the bone marrow. The iron binding saturation is a more reliable index; levels of 16% or below are not found when there are more traces of iron in the bone marrow,[8] though higher saturations may on occasion accompany undoubted iron deficiency.

The mean cell haemoglobin and the blood film should always be taken into account.

As many as 10 % of elderly people living at home have an abnormally low iron binding saturation but a normal haemoglobin concentration and a normal blood film.[4] Women of reproductive age who show this picture of "sideropenia without anaemia" have a high chance of developing frank iron deficiency anaemia within a few years,[9] but whether the same is true of the elderly is not known. There is at present no reason to treat them since no symptomatic benefit accrues.[9,10]

Folate and B_{12} concentrations

The serum folate has been largely superseded by the red cell content, for which the customary lower limit of normal of 120 nmol/l of red cells should be taken. Confident statements about the frequency of folate deficiency in the elderly need to be reinterpreted in the light of this latter test.

A low serum vitamin B_{12} concentration (below 140 pmol/l) can be taken to indicate deficiency of that vitamin as a cause of a megaloblastic anaemia in an old person, but low concentrations are also commonly encountered in elderly people without anaemia, macrocytosis, or disorder of the nervous system.[4] It is not yet known how frequently or how soon overt clinical disease may be expected to develop in such people, who may perhaps still possess hepatic stores of vitamin B_{12} sufficient to last for long periods, but they are not symptomatically benefited from therapy with vitamin B_{12}.[11]

White cell count

The white cell count tends to fall with age, mainly owing to a reduction in lymphocyte count.[12] The upper limit of normal for the total white cell count is $9 \times 10^9/l$[13,14] – that is, less than the textbook figure of $10–11 \times 10^9/l$. Total counts over $9 \times 10^9/l$ may thus be taken to indicate leucocytosis. The lower limit of the total count is $3 \times 10^9/l$, and leucopenia should therefore not be diagnosed unless the count is below this figure, rather than the customary concentrations of $4–5 \times 10^9/l$.

Erythrocyte sedimentation rate (ESR)

Some uncertainty surrounds the interpretation of the ESR in old age. Studies to determine the true normal limits of this valuable simple test are difficult to carry out in the elderly since even after the exclusion of acutely ill subjects, who will constitute a high proportion of any hospital series, there remain many old people with chronic conditions associated with a raised ESR. Undoubtedly mean values rise steadily with age in healthy people and are higher in women than men[15]; it is also clear that no convincing cause may be found in old people for values as high as 30–35 mm in the first hour.[2] As in younger people, the isolated finding of a raised ESR is best repeated after a few weeks, and only a persistent rise outside the limits mentioned should be regarded as an indication for further investigation.

Biochemical tests

In many commonly performed biochemical tests mean normal values and the range encountered in relatively healthy old people are identical to those found in the young (table I[14,16]). Abnormalities in these cannot therefore be attributed to aging but require

TABLE I – *Normal values for biochemical measurements in old age*[16]

Substance	Mean	SD	Range
Na⁺ (mmol/l)	141	3	136–146
K⁺ (mmol/l)	4.4	0.4	3·6–5.2
Cl⁻ (mmol/l)	102	3	96–108
HCO₃⁻ (mmol/l)	25	3	19–31
Total			
Protein (g/l)	71	5	61–81
Albumin (g/l)	41	4	34–50
Globulin (g/l)	31	5	21–41
Mg⁺⁺ (mmol/l)	0.82	0.1	0.62–1.02
PO₄⁻⁻ (mmol)			
Men	1.00	0.16	0.65–1.27
Women	1.05	0.19	0.68–1.43
Bilirubin (mmol/l)		*	5–26

* Log normal frequency distribution.
Conversion: SI to traditional units – Sodium: 1 mmol = 1 mEq.
Potassium: 1 mmol = 1 mEq. Chloride: 1 mmol = 1 mEq.
Magnesium: 1 mmol ≈ 2.4 mg/100 ml. Phosphate: 1 mmol ≈ 31 mg.
Bilirubin: 1 mmol/l ≈ 58.5 mg/100 ml.

assessment and diagnosis. The abnormalities most frequently met with are hypokalaemia, of which the commonest cause is diuretic drugs, and hypoalbuminaemia, which may be due to chronic infection, malignancy, diffuse liver disease, or rarely to simple malnutrition, which should never be presumed to be the cause of hypoalbuminaemia without further investigation. The criteria for the identification of these abnormalities, and the action which should follow their detection, do not differ in essence in old age from standard practice in younger patients.

Blood urea and creatinine

For a second group of measurements the range of normal values is not the same in the elderly as in the young (table II). The differences are relatively small but none the less important. The

TABLE II – *Normal values which differ in old age*[16]

Substance	Mean	SD	Range
Urea (mmol/l)	★		4–10
Creatinine (μmol/l)	★		35–170
Cholesterol (mmol/l)			
Men	★		4.2–9.0
Women	★		4.7–11.3
Ca^{++} (mmol/l)			
Men	2.40	0.13	2.20–2.60
Women	2.50	0.13	2.30–2.70
Uric acid (mmol/l)			
Men	0.33	0.07	0.19–0.47
Women	0.29	0.08	0.13–0.46

★ Log normal frequency distribution.
Conversion: SI to traditional units – Urea: 1 mmol/l ≈ 6 mg/100 ml.
Creatinine: 1 μmol/l ≈ 11 μg/100 ml. Cholesterol: 1 mmol/l ≈ 39 mg/100 ml.
Calcium: 1 mmol/l ≈ 4 mg/100 ml. Urate: 1 mmol/l ≈ 16.8 mg/100 ml.

most obvious example is the blood urea concentration, which is the result of the urea production and the glomerular filtration rates. The former probably falls with age, and the latter certainly does[17] and to a greater extent, so that the plasma concentration of urea rises with age.[16] The upper limit of normal for the blood urea concentration in people over 65 is about 10 mmol/l (60 mg/100 ml). Renal failure, with its poor prognosis and attendant potentially hazardous investigations, should not be diagnosed if the blood urea value is below this figure. Exactly similar considerations apply to the serum creatinine,[18] for which a reasonable upper limit of normal in old age is 170 μmol/l (1.9 mg/100 ml), rather than the customary figure of 130 μmol/l (1.5 mg/100 ml).

Uric acid, cholesterol, and calcium concentrations

There is undoubtedly an age related rise in the serum uric acid value. Concentrations below 0.46 mmol/l should be regarded as normal and cannot be used to support a diagnosis of gout in an old person. The thiazide diuretics are the commonest cause of an increased serum uric acid level in old age.

The serum cholesterol concentration rises with age and after the menopause is higher in women than in men, the reverse of the situation below that age. There may well be considerable local variation in normal concentrations in old age,[14,16] associated with nutritional differences, but in urban Scotland over 40% of women and 8% of men over the age of 65 have a serum cholesterol concentration of over 7.8 mmol/l (304 mg/100 ml).[16] These high values are not associated with coronary artery disease, or with hypothyroidism, and only very high figures (of over 11.7 mmol/l (456 mg/100 ml) or so) can be used to support the latter diagnosis in an old person. There is as yet no convincing evidence that lowering the serum cholesterol is of benefit to an elderly patient.

A further example of a normal range which may differ in old people is the serum calcium concentration. In elderly women the commonly accepted upper limit of 2.5 mmol/l (10 mg/100 ml) seems too low,[16] and values of 2.7 or even 2.8 mmol/l (10.8 or 11.2 mg/100 ml) may be found in the absence of other biochemical or radiological evidence of hyperparathyroidism (although this commonly may be entirely asymptomatic in old age[19]) or any other cause of hypercalcaemia. The sex difference shown in table II for serum calcium may perhaps be of clinical importance.

Phosphatases

It is uncertain whether the normal range of serum alkaline phosphatase is the same in young and old. A rise in mean values with age has long been attributed to an age related increase in the prevalence of Paget's disease, and more recently to osteomalacia since the recognition that this disorder is common in elderly women.[32] Nevertheless, in elderly hospital patients osteomalacia and Paget's disease are considerably less frequent conditions associated with a serum alkaline phosphatase activity above the conventional upper limit of normality of 350 IU/l than are liver disease, recent bone trauma, or malignant secondary deposits. At present it would seem reasonable to regard a serum alkaline phosphatase activity of over perhaps 400 IU/l as abnormal in an old person, and an indication for a search for liver or bone disease, and a value between 350 and 400 IU/l as of uncertain significance. Values of over 1000 IU/l will usually be found to be due to Paget's disease, either obvious clinically or detectable on a relatively restricted set of radiographs (for example, of the chest and pelvis), or to metastatic liver disease, of which there may be little other biochemical evidence. Determination of the isoenzymes of alkaline phosphatase is of great value in distinguishing between raised activities due to bone disease and those due to hepatic disease.

Normal values for serum acid phosphatase are the same in the elderly as in middle age, and measurement of the tartrate-labile fraction is of great value in the diagnosis and management of prostatic carcinoma, one of the controllable cancers. There is no evidence for any age related difference in the concentrations of other commonly estimated serum enzymes, such as aspartate or alanine transferase[14,20]; the upper limit of normal of lactic dehydrogenase may be as high as 225 IU/l.[14]

Tests of endocrine function

The endocrine disorders common in old age are diabetes mellitus, hyperthyroidism, and hypothyroidism. All others are distinctly rare, and only those tests relevant to the three common conditions mentioned will be discussed.

Diabetes

The most important single measurement in the diagnosis of diabetes is the random blood sugar concentration. Values below 8 mmol/l (144 mg/100 ml) may be accepted as normal in the elderly and values over 11 mmol/l (198 mg/100 ml) as indicative of diabetes – and thus requiring appropriate treatment.[21] Most old people with blood sugar concentrations over 11 mmol/l have glycosuria, and many have frank diabetic symptoms – though these may only come to light on direct questioning. Consideration of all the circumstances, including the presence or absence of symptoms, repetition of the random blood sugar, measurement or HbA_1[20], or determination of the fasting blood sugar (a value of 8 mmol/l or more indicating diabetes) will help in deciding whether a diagnosis of diabetes and all it entails is justified. A glucose tolerance test may only increase the uncertainties. Many old people have "impaired glucose tolerance" as defined,[8] with a blood glucose two hours after oral glucose of between 7 mmol/l (126 mg/100 ml) (the figure defining normality) and 11 mmol/l (the figure defining diabetes). Their chance of developing diabetes is somewhat greater than normal but they do not warrant active treatment.

Thyroid disease

Of the numerous tests for thyroid function, those using only blood samples have much to recommend them in the diagnosis of thyroid disease in the elderly. Age alone produces only very minor effects on thyroid hormone concentrations, once the common occurrence of overt thyroid disease has been excluded.[23] Both acute illness and therapy with a wide variety of drugs may result in complex disturbances of thyroxine output, protein binding, and metabolism,[24] with consequent disturbance of hormone estimations. In general these tests should be delayed until or repeated after the acute illness is over, as interpretation then becomes easier. Of particular importance are high or low values of total thyroxine and tri-iodothyronine, which cannot be entirely corrected for by the use of the free thyroxine index. Direct measurement of free thyroxine concentrations (only 0.3% of the total) may help.[25]

Raised concentrations of thyroid stimulating hormone (above 11 IU/l) are virtually diagnostic of primary (but not of secondary pituitary) hypothyroidism, while a fall to normal will confirm the adequacy of thyroid replacement therapy.

Conclusion

Laboratory investigations are essential for the accurate diagnosis of many treatable conditions common in the elderly. The proper interpretation of the results of such investigations demands a knowledge both of the normal values encountered in old age and of the numerous factors which may produce misleading results.

[1] Chalmers DG, Myers AM, Saunders CRG. The haemoglobin level of fit elderly people. *Lancet* 1968; ii: 261–3.
[2] Landahl S, Jagenburg R, Svanborg A. Blood components in a 70-year old population. *Clin Chim Acta* 1981; **112**: 301–14.
[3] World Health Organisation. *Nutritional Anaemias*. Geneva: WHO, 1968. (WHO Technical Report Series No 405.)
[4] McLennan WJ, Andrews GR, Caird FI, MacLeod CC. Anaemia in the elderly. *Q J Med* 1973; **43**: 1–14.
[5] Powell DEB, Thomas JH. *Blood disorders in the elderly*. Bristol: J Wright, 1971.
[6] Wu A, Chanarin I, Levi AJ. Macrocytosis of chronic alcoholism. *Lancet* 1974; i: 829–31.
[7] Bothwell TH, Finch CA. *Iron metabolism*. Boston: Little Brown, 1962.
[8] Bainton DF, Finch CA. The diagnosis of iron deficiency anemia. *Am J Med* 1964; **37**: 62–70.
[9] Dagg JH, Goldberg A, Morrow JJ. A controlled trial of iron therapy in sideropenia. *Scott Med J* 1968; **13**: 78–83.
[10] Elwood PC, Hughes D. Clinical trial of iron therapy on psychomotor function in anaemic women. *Br Med J* 1970; iii: 254–5.
[11] Elwood PC, Hughes D, Shinton NK, Wrighton RJ. Clinical trial of the effect of vitamin B_{12} in elderly subjects with low serum B12 levels. *Br Med J* 1970; ii: 458–60.
[12] McKinney AA. Effect of aging on the peripheral blood lymphocyte count. *J Gerontol* 1980; **33**: 213–6.
[13] Caird FI, Andrews GR, Gallie TB. The leucocyte count in old age. *Age Ageing* 1972; **1**: 239–44.

[14] Hale WE, Stewart RB, Marks RG. Haematological and biochemical laboratory values in an ambulant elderly population: an analysis of the effects of age, sex, and drugs. *Age Ageing* 1983; **12**: 275–84.

[15] Bottiger LE, Svedberg CA. Normal erythrocyte sedimentation rate and age. *Br Med J* 1967; ii: 85–7.

[16] Leask RGS, Andrews GR, Caird FI. Normal values for sixteen blood constituents in the elderly. *Age Ageing* 1973; ii: 14–23.

[17] Rowe JW. Renal system. In: Rowe JW, Besdine RW, eds. *Health and disease in old age*. Boston: Little Brown, 1982: 165–83.

[18] Pearson MW. Asymptomatic hyperparathyroidism in the elderly – a review. *Age Ageing* 1984; **13**: 1–5.

[19] Kampman JP, Sinding J, Moller-Jorgensen I. Effect of age on liver function. *Geriatrics* 1975; **30**: 91–5.

[20] Martin BJ, Knight PV, Kesson CM, O'Donnell JR, Young RE. Glycosylated haemoglobin: its value in screening for diabetes in the elderly. *J Clin Exp Gerontol* 1984; **6**: 87–94.

[21] WHO Expert Committee on Diabetes Mellitus. *Second report*. Geneva: WHO, 1980. (WHO Technical Report Series No 646.)

[22] Evered DC, Tunbridge WMG, Hall R, *et al*. Thyroid hormone concentrations in a large scale community survey. Effect of age, sex, illness, and medication. *Clin Chim Acta* 1978; **83**: 223–9.

[23] Thomson JA. Thyroid function. In: Exton-Smith AN, Caird FI, eds. *Metabolic and nutritional disorders in the elderly*. Bristol: J Wright, 1980: 199–210.

[24] Crowe MJ, Gales M, Griffiths RA, Moore RA, Wollner L. Free thyroxine measurements in elderly patients with suspected hypothyroidism. *J Clin Exp Gerontol* 1984; **6**: 173–86.

Mental disturbance in ill, old people

TOM DUNN AND TOM ARIE

Mental disturbance is common in ill old people and the mortality in this group is high. Management can be difficult, and mismanagement can change a restless ill patient into an apathetic, dehydrated, incontinent patient with pressure sores, at grave risk of dying from pneumonia or pulmonary emboli. Serious problems arise from acute confusional states and from severe depression, but paranoid states and hypomania can also be troublesome.

Acute confusional states

Some degree of mental impairment is a common accompaniment of aging; even when there is frank dementia many, at least in the earlier years, remain sufficiently competent to go on living in a simpler way with their families or even by themselves. Physical illness or other adverse factors in aged, and especially very aged, people can readily cause acute confusion and precipitate a domestic crisis. Even when there is no obvious mental impairment the aged brain tends to have less "reserve," so that it is much more readily upset than the younger brain by drugs or illness. As a result more than a third of all patients admitted directly to geriatric departments are confused.

The mental symptoms may range from mild delirium to restless, agitated, and aggressive behaviour, sometimes with hallucinations and paranoid delusions. Many patients are obviously physically ill, but in some the psychiatric symptoms dominate the picture.

Commoner causes of confusional states

Strokes

Patients with strokes causing major paralysis may also be confused, but the cause is obvious. However, the area of cerebral infarction may not involve the pyramidal tracts, and the problem may then present as acute confusion. Careful examination may detect some confirmatory signs such as minor weakness or clumsiness of a limb or an extensor plantar response. Examination should include rough tests of the visual fields as homonymous hemianopia is easily missed in a confused person. Its presence contributes to the confusion but also may confirm that there has been a stroke.

A stroke may present only with dysphasia, or with jargon dysphasia, so that the patient's speech is gibberish. Such a patient may be confused or may only appear to be confused because of the nonsensical speech. Examination will reveal nominal dysphasia, and sensible behaviour may be out of keeping with the disturbed speech. These disabilities can be frightening and bewildering to the patient, who may become agitated and frustrated, and this can add to the difficulty of diagnosis. Dyspraxias and agnosias are commonly mistaken for "confusion."

At the onset of the stroke there may be headache, vomiting, vertigo, or ataxia as well as the acute onset of confusion. In many cases, however, there will be no confirmatory signs and one is left with a presumptive diagnosis based on the history of sudden onset and on the exclusion of other factors. Whether further neurological investigation, such as computed tomography, is justified depends on the course and on local facilities. As with paralysis there is a natural tendency for the confusional state to improve with time, though further strokes are common.

Cerebral ischaemia

There are many causes of cerebral ischaemia, without actual infarction, which can cause confusion. Low cardiac output may be due to congestive heart failure, cardiac infarction, or pulmonary emboli or associated with abdominal emergencies such as volvulus, mesenteric infarction, or gastrointestinal bleeding.

Cerebral hypoxia

Patients with chronic respiratory failure readily become confused, especially with infection or with the onset of cor pulmonale, but may become lucid again as the acute episode subsides. Chronic anaemias cause confusion only when they are quite severe, with haemoglobin concentrations usually below 6.0 g/dl. Confusion may occur in vitamin B_{12} deficiency states even without anaemia but only rarely responds to vitamin B_{12} injections.

Subdural haematoma

Though subdural haematoma is uncommon, it can be rewarding to find and disastrous to miss. Fortunately, diagnosis is usually simple with the help of computed tomography. Subdural haematoma must be suspected when there is a history of falls and when confusion or consciousness is fluctuant. Old people with friable atheromatous vessels are particularly at risk, and there may be no clear history of trauma. Sometimes acute symptoms turn out to be associated with very old haematomas or hygromas, and even here the results of surgery can be excellent.

A prominent local citizen of 67 had been noticed to be progressively behaving more oddly over several months, a development which was attributed to his well known fondness of alcohol. When he became acutely confused and aggressive one Saturday night, the psychiatrist was summoned with a view to compulsory hospitalisation. There was papilloedema and minimal long tract signs, and bilateral subdural hygromas of apparently very long standing were evacuated that night. He remained very confused for several weeks after operation, but subsequently returned to full normality, with no detectable intellectual deficits: and was very well two years later.

Cerebral tumour

A change in the behaviour and personality over a period of weeks or months may be the first evidence of cerebral tumour, either primary or secondary. When suspicion is aroused either by the history or by associated signs investigation, such as computed tomography, will be required; often in this age group it is not reasonable to undertake surgery, but in some patients, even the very old, surgery may be followed by worthwhile, and even dramatic, improvement especially for benign tumours such as meningiomas and acoustic neuromas.

Myxoedema

The mental symptoms of myxoedema are usually lethargy and slowing of thought processes. Occasionally there may be confusion or a depressive or paranoid picture – the "myxoedematous madness" of Richard Asher. This may respond slowly to small doses of thyroxine; in most cases, however, the mental state is not improved, though the general physical state will be.

Diabetes

Diabetic hyperglycaemia or acidosis may present with confusion as well as drowsiness. More frequent, and much more important, is the confusional state due to iatrogenic hypoglycaemia, especially from oral antidiabetic drugs. Diabetes is common in old people, and many are unnecessarily started on oral drugs when the mild diabetes could be controlled by diet only. The hypoglycaemia may be far from obvious as it often presents as a confusional state without sweating or hypotension. It may come on insidiously and persist for hours or even for days if the treatment is continued. It should always be suspected when there is confused behaviour in someone on oral hypoglycaemic drugs. Confirmation is easy from a stick blood test, but if there is doubt the diagnosis is confirmed by the brisk therapeutic response to oral carbohydrate or to 25 g of intravenous glucose. The hypoglycaemia may recur over the next 24 hours. Chlorpropamide is not the drug of first choice in the elderly because its long action makes hypoglycaemia particularly dangerous, and it is generally better to use one of the many shorter acting sulphonylureas as the first choice. Chronic brain failure is common in diabetes, probably because of increased prevalence of atheroma, but sometimes because of past cerebral damage from severe hypoglycaemia.

Toxic causes

Infections – In a young person pneumonia can cause delirium, but in older people this may follow less severe infections. In old people infections – for example, pneumonia or urinary infections – can be silent till they are quite advanced and a change in the mental state may be the presenting symptom.

Tissue necrosis – A patient ill and confused with gangrene of a leg may be much improved after amputation. In the same way a major pressure sore adds to the gravity of the illness of the patient already ill enough to develop a sore. Absorption of blood, either from a large haematoma which may accompany a fracture of the femur or from the gut after gastrointestinal haemorrhage, may exacerbate both the physical and the mental disturbance.

Other toxic causes – Chronic renal failure is fairly common and, with the associated anaemia, can make the patient ill and confused, but some patients manage reasonably well until there is some infection or other illness, when the patient quickly becomes ill and confused. Renal failure greatly increases the risk of toxicity from drugs – for example, digoxin. Even healthy elderly people have less renal reserve so that they more readily develop prerenal uraemia from an inadequate fluid intake. Electrolyte imbalance may be due to fluid or electrolyte loss; to renal failure or the effect of drugs; or to a combination of these factors and, whatever the cause, may contribute to the illness and to a confusional state.

Drugs

It is natural that older people have more complaints than younger people, and it is all too easy to give a drug for each one: for example, for hypertension – a β blocker; for giddiness – prochlorperazine; for ankle oedema, irrespective of cause – a diuretic; for anxiety – a tranquilliser; and so on.

Old people's brains are more easily befuddled and they are often subjected to greater concentrations of drugs, partly because of the number of drugs prescribed, partly because a degree of renal failure impairs excretion, partly through other changes in drug handling by the aging body, and partly because so often a "frail lady" has such a small body mass. It is important to avoid overtreating elderly people. Time after time we have seen a remarkable improvement in the physical and mental state when all the numerous drugs have been stopped. If the elderly patient is on a complicated regimen it is virtually certain that the regimen will not be properly followed, and it may be the important drugs that are omitted. This is likely to make evaluation even more difficult because one can never be certain what the patient is actually taking. It should seldom be necessary to prescribe more than three different regular drugs. The recent report from the Royal College of Physicians of London (1984) on medication in the elderly gives sensible advice on these matters.

The drugs which are most likely to precipitate confusion are those which act directly on the nervous system, and the most notorious are the antiparkinsonian drugs.

A patient was admitted in a confused agitated state, tottery, and having had some falls. Over the next day or two he returned to his normal slightly forgetful self and after returning home to his elderly wife he remained well for a week. He then again became acutely confused and that night fell on getting out of bed and was incontinent of faeces. This crisis precipitated a home visit next day, when a bottle of benzhexol tablets was found. Inquiry revealed that they had been started just before the first admission but had not been resumed after discharge till the previous day, when his wife asked the district nurse if she should restart them. One tablet was apparently enough to cause this crisis.

All the anticholinergic drugs as well as levodopa, bromocriptine, and amantadine can cause insomnia, restlessness, hallucinations,

129

and delusions. These drugs must be started in small doses and built up gradually and should not be pressed to the concentrations used in younger people.

The advertisement picture of a "tranquillised" old lady entertaining a party at the piano has generally not been our experience. All sedatives and tranquillisers are likely to make an ill old person bemused and lethargic and add to the difficulties of nursing care. They can also cause hypotension with fainting or falls and can contribute to hypothermia. They may be necessary to control restlessness or delusions, but when they must be prescribed the starting dose should be less than in younger people. Hypnotics too increase the susceptibility to falls during the night and may cause nocturnal confusion. It is hardly ever necessary for old people to have hypnotics regularly. When prescribed for a single occasion or for a short spell the dose should be lower than in younger people whatever hypnotic is used.

Antidepressants are valuable but can cause excitement and confusion. Monoamine oxidase inhibitors are only rarely appropriate for old people and should not be initiated by the general practitioner. Finally, one must not forget that elderly as well as younger people may be alcoholics, with ataxia and a chronic befuddled state.

Other drugs not normally associated with action on the central nervous system can cause confusion, and some examples are toxic doses of digoxin, therapeutic doses of cimetidine or ranitidine, and the higher doses of steroids.

Epilepsy

In addition to longstanding idiopathic epilepsy, new cases of epilepsy are common, mostly due to vascular brain damage. The seizures may be followed by a period of drowsy confusion but are often atypical and may present as transient episodes of confused behaviour. In the elderly the doses of antiepileptic drugs used in younger people may cause unsteadiness and confusion.

Multiple factors

Often it is not possible to point to a single cause of confusion in an ill, old person. It may be due partly to the primary illness; partly to removal from familiar surroundings; partly to dehydration or electrolyte disturbance; partly to the drugs used; and to complications such as venous thrombosis or pressure sores.

Principles of diagnosis and management

Diagnosis

It is important to obtain a full history of the development of the illness and this must include a history from a relative, friend, or neighbour. It is very important to ascertain what was the mental state of the patient *before* the illness. The abrupt onset of confusion suggests the possibility of a stroke. The development of confused behaviour over some weeks or months in a previously normal person raises the possibility of a cerebral tumour. A history of previous mental illness – for example, depression – even many years ago, may be a valuable clue.

An 82 year old woman, looking very deteriorated, virtually mute, and incontinent and refusing food and drink was admitted to our joint unit. The recent history was not clear, but a relatively sudden deterioration seemed to have occurred. The family said there was no previous history of psychiatric illness. The woman looked sad, and the nursing staff were asked to keep a careful record of the few utterances she made. These turned out to be almost all self disparaging, and depression was tentatively diagnosed. Despite general supportive measures she continued to decline, and so was given electroconvulsive therapy, to which she made a steady and gratifying response. It was only at this point that the family "confessed" that she had had an almost identical illness 20 years ago, when she had likewise recovered after electroconvulsive therapy.

The inquiry must include a drug history and especially the relation of the onset of confusion to any new therapy. Physical examination may be difficult but must not be neglected and should include neurological examination.

The cause of the illness and the mental disturbance will often then be clear, and if the facilities are adequate the patient can be managed at home; where the cause is not clear, the advice of a geriatric physician or psychiatrist should be sought at a domiciliary consultation. When the cause cannot be established at home, or when sufficient facilities, or tolerance, to nurse the patient at home are not available, the patient must be admitted to hospital. Because the accent will normally be on physical investigations and general nursing care, admission should be sought not to a psychiatric department but to the geriatric or medical department. Where there are beds jointly cared for by a psychiatrist and the geriatrician within the geriatric department admission to this unit will then often be best.

Management

The management of an ill confused old person is one of the most difficult problems in the practice of medicine. Every effort must be made to find and treat the underlying cause or causes, not just to treat the mental disturbance symptomatically. While waiting for treatment to take effect or for natural recovery symptomatic and supportive treatment will be necessary.

If the patient is restless sedation will probably be required, but strong sedation is likely to add to the gravity of the primary illness. If the patient is ambulant sedation will make her liable to fall. If sedation is sufficient to keep her in bed it is likely to lead to pressure sores, venous thrombosis, or serious dehydration. Even without sedation it may be difficult to get adequate fluids into ill confused patients (a careful record should always be kept of fluid intake and, as far as possible, of output).

For these reasons the least possible sedation should be used. The more nursing time that can be devoted to the patient the less will be the need for sedatives and the easier it will be to maintain an adequate fluid intake. Where there is a willing relative this will be best achieved at home; moreover, the patient may be less disorientated in his own surroundings and with his own family. Reassurance, familiar attendants, and, in hospital, minimum change of surroundings are all as important as sedative drugs. Good lighting can be important; some patients become much more confused in shadowy, ill lit rooms. Disturbed behaviour is apt to be worse at night and more distressing to relatives, who themselves become irritable through chronic lack of sleep; so hypnotics will usually be required. Chloral should not be forgotten – for example, as dichloralphenazone. The most popular hypnotics in geriatric practice, however, are the shorter acting benzodiazepines, such as temazepam or triazolam; of the medium duration drugs, lormetazepam has also been found useful. The danger with longer acting drugs such as nitrazepam is that they are cumulative and if used for more than one night may cause day time "doping." Chlormethiazole is short acting and effective but does not suit everyone. Occasionally in very restless patients a combination of a phenothiazine – for example, promazine 25 mg and dichloralphenazone – may help, but such combinations need to be used with care: over sedation may result not only in hangovers but in falls. Where restlessness is a problem by day, regular phenothiazine drugs may be required if the restlessness cannot be controlled by the family or nursing staff. In old and frail people it is probably better to use promazine – for example, 25 mg up to three times a day – rather than the stronger chlorpromazine because the dose of the weaker drug may be more exactly adjusted; and chlorpromazine jaundice is common. Such drugs are cumulative, and the effect increases over the first day or two when the dose may have to be reduced.

There is much to be said for the doctor relying on one or two major tranquillisers with which he is familiar, rather than trying out the latest one. Long acting injected tranquillisers in oily solution are best avoided in frail old people because once injected their dosage cannot be regulated and side effects can be very troublesome. A wild and aggressive patient who cannot be calmed may need more dramatic action. Chlorpromazine 50 mg by injection will usually be effective, but this should be a single dose and not repeated regularly without reassessment. When the patient cannot be controlled by these means, or where dehydration threatens to become a problem, admission to hospital will be needed. It may then be necessary to rehydrate the patient by giving quite heavy sedation so that she will not interfere with a stomach tube or intravenous or other parenteral infusion.

There is no good evidence for giving massive doses of vitamins to confused patients. It is reasonable to give vitamins in therapeutic doses to those patients who have been living in a state of neglect and malnutrition, and of course especially if alcoholism is known or suspected. Search for bottles should be part of the routine assessment of the elderly recluse or isolate.

Depression

Depression in old people may respond excellently to drug treatment or to electroconvulsive therapy, and lithium can be most useful. But diagnosis may be difficult; and physical treatments call for special care. Depression in old age may present with physical complaints, or as confusion – without primarily depressive features. A history of depression can be a crucial clue. The patient may be agitated, or withdrawn and even mute. She may refuse food and drink, so that she becomes dehydrated and seriously ill. Suicide is always a risk, being commoner in the aged. Sometimes the patient is befuddled, and the picture may be of a confusional state; at other times there is a preoccupation with loss of memory and the picture may resemble dementia ("pseudodementia"); but truly demented patients rarely parade their forgetfulness.

Such patients may need careful psychiatric appraisal. In largely mute or confused patients nurses should record any coherent talk, which may be depressive in nature. These patients may be at risk from physical deterioration, especially from dehydration and metabolic derangement, and a joint medical/psychiatric unit may be the best place for their care – or a joint department of physicians and psychiatrists such as exists in Nottingham.

A 68 year old man "collapsed" whilst visiting his wife, who had for many years been a patient in a mental hospital. He was himself admitted to hospital, but despite extensive investigations no physical cause for his "collapse" was found; but he was withdrawn, refused food, and looked sad. It turned out that his dog, with whom he had lived alone for many years since his wife's hospitalisation, had recently died, and his neighbours had noticed that he had initially stopped going out. A diagnosis of depression was made, though some degree of dementia was also suspected. Treatment with amitriptyline was started, but he became very dehydrated and was transferred to a geriatric unit. He became grossly confused, withdrawn, and ill. He was rehydrated, and intercurrent chest infection was treated, and he was given electroconvulsive therapy, whereupon he recovered to full normality with no signs of intellectual impairment; and six months later wrote a long and impeccable letter reporting his progress, having moved to another part of the country, to which he wished also be bring his wife.

Paranoid states

Chronic delusional states without progressive dementia, usually paranoid, are not uncommon in old people. They often live with their delusions, though they may cause concern to others. With new physical illness the delusional state may become more severe or come to the notice of the doctor for the first time. Persecutory states often respond to phenothiazine or butyrophenone treatment, sometimes dramatically, but it is often difficult to persuade the patients to continue to take their drugs, especially if they are living alone.

Hypomania

Hypomania is much less common than depression but is not rare in old age. Cerebral disease seems often to be the trigger. The patient may be agitated, restless, talking incessantly, sometimes confused. She may be euphoric, or there may be a paradoxical admixture of depression. If overactive she may become quite ill. The hypomanic episode usually responds to tranquillisers or lithium (renal function must be carefully checked before using the latter).

Conclusion

Mental disturbances in ill old people are life threatening, but with careful diagnosis and treatment the outlook (depending on the causes) may be excellent. Such patients need expert and painstaking attention.

Diet in the elderly

D CORLESS

The King Edward's Hospital Fund's 1965 report of an investigation into the diet of elderly women living alone stated, "the precise nutritional needs of old people are unknown."[1] Nearly 20 years later this statement is as true as it was then. More sophisticated investigatory techniques yield more knowledge but frequently increase the areas of doubt, for example, the ability developed during the last 20 years to measure vitamin D metabolites (see below). Opinions vary widely about the incidence of malnutrition,[2] particularly if subclinical disease is sought. Not surprisingly the incidence depends on the type of person investigated; it is lower in healthy people living at home than in enfeebled people in institutions. Geography has an effect through social conditions, and the amount of sunlight and racial factors may also influence the incidence.

The ideal diet

Homo sapiens, thought to be omnivorous by the design of his dentition, can live healthily on a vegetarian diet, though strict vegetarians are prone to vitamin B_{12} deficiency. A vegetarian diet, carefully formulated, approaches the ideal for longevity. Carbohydrates in a rapidly absorbable, often highly refined, form predispose to diabetes mellitus, but the presence of vegetable dietary fibre reduces the speed of absorption of carbohydrates. Fibre prevents constipation and reduces the risk of diverticulitis. Prevention of coronary vascular disease can be accomplished by diets high in polyunsaturated fats, usually of vegetable origin. Meat eaters have a diet high in cholesterol and are at risk of atheroma, though fish oil containing unsaturated eicosapentaenoic acid protects Eskimos from this disease. Eating meat is also associated with a higher risk of bowel cancer.

Dietary recommendations

Carbohydrate	Emphasis on unrefined, high fibre, slowly absorbed forms
Dietary fibre	25–30 g/day. Sources are beans, lentils, wholemeal bread, vegetables (including potatoes)
Sucrose	Ideally absent from diet, but less than 35 g/day added as sugar, and less than 75 g/day contained in foods (cakes, pastry, etc)
Protein	More than 10% of total energy intake ($\geqslant$ 58 g/day)
Fat	Less than 35 g/day with high content of polyunsaturated fats (remove visible fat from meat)
Minerals	
Potassium	Fresh fruit and fruit juice, salad, vegetables
Salt	No added salt, minimum necessary for cooking (usual diet contains > 20 × physiological requirement)
Vitamins	
Vitamin A	5000 IU
Vitamin B$_1$ (*thiamine*)	0.8 mg
Vitamin B$_2$ (*riboflavine*)	1.3 mg
Vitamin B$_{12}$	5 μg
Folic acid	0.25 mg
Vitamin C	30 mg★
Vitamin D	400 IU (10 μg)★

★ DHSS recommended daily amounts, 1979.

A high salt intake is associated with hypertension; a reduced salt intake is beneficial (see table).

Dietary measures designed to prevent many of the illnesses complicating old age should be adopted at an early stage of life. This in itself raises the doubt that such recommendations have not yet been tested by long term trials. Even the common recommendation to ensure a diet with "adequate" amounts of calcium and vitamin D to prevent osteoporosis and the serious complication of fracture of the proximal femur has not yet been so validated.

Diet in old age

Even accepting these caveats certain guidelines for a diet suitable for old people can be given.[3] Fit elderly people are notable for a high energy intake, and longitudinal studies have shown that these "elite" elderly maintain their high energy intakes with advancing age.[4] In fact the often quoted "normal" decline in dietary intake with increasing age is based on cross sectional studies; much of the decline can be caused by clinical and subclinical illness. Lean body mass diminishes with age, which slightly reduces the need for energy intake, but the major determinant is energy expenditure, which tends to fall with age. The diet should provide enough energy to maintain body weight with normal physical activity. Disabled people who walk inefficiently may expend surprisingly high amounts of energy and need high energy diets.

Overnutrition results in obesity, and the obese may suffer the principal complications of hypertension, diabetes, and skeletal problems. Weight reduction by dieting is often an important part of rehabilitation. Obese old people and those who are immobile need less energy than expected, and a reducing diet may have to be apparently severe, even less than 2.5 MJ (600 kcal), for good effect. The obese can suffer malnutrition, often due to a poorly formulated reducing diet.

The usual amount of protein in the diet is 10% or more of the total intake (about 58 g/day). The high energy intake of the elite group contains in excess of 70 g protein per day.

Carbohydrates make up most of the energy intake and are the cheapest form of energy. Their proportion of the diet increases as poverty occurs and the percentage protein intake falls below 10%.

Minimal needs of vitamins and minerals are shown in the table and mentioned in the text.

Aetiological factors in malnutrition

Nutrition considered in isolation is an intellectual abstraction. Eating is not solely to sustain life; the preparation and consumption of food is done with others for enjoyment. Thus social isolation due to bereavement or families living far away may be major factors in malnutrition. Depression may be responsible for much self neglect and presents atypically in the elderly, often by physical symptoms alone, or with "pseudodementia." Increasing physical infirmity leads to problems in shopping and cooking, compounded by poor housing and the isolation of houses from shops. Retirement to "a place near the sea" often brings unexpected difficulties when infirmities develop.

Illness in old age often leads to an inadequate diet, and it is important to remember that diseases may present with non-specific symptoms such as confusion, incontinence, or falls. Multiple pathology is frequent and makes diagnosis more difficult. The anorexic old person "failing to thrive" may well have an occult illness such as apathetic thyrotoxicosis, tuberculosis, acute rheumatoid arthritis, malignancy, etc; examination and investigation need to be humanely thorough.

Gastrointestinal disease is common in the elderly and malabsorption is often asymptomatic. Jejunal diverticula or blind loops may be found in patients with osteomalacia or vitamin B_{12} or folic acid deficiency. Idiopathic steatorrhoea can first present in old age.

Drugs present an additional nutritional hazard, and it is well known that barbiturates and anticonvulsants lead to folic acid deficiency. They also cause osteomalacia by creating target organ resistance to vitamin D.

Long stay patients in institutions are often deprived of sunlight and have diets low in vitamin D, calcium, iron, vitamin C, and folic acid; osteomalacia, scurvy, and anaemia are some of the complications faced by the inmates.[5]

Clinical presentation

Deficiency states are usually compound problems; thus iron and folic acid deficiency, scurvy, and osteomalacia may occur together. The deficiencies described are restricted to those found commonly in geriatric practice, and a text book approach is used for convenience, each deficiency being considered separately.

Protein deficiency

A lowered intake of protein leads to loss of body weight; equilibrium may be reached when the consequent weakness reduces energy expenditure. Severe protein lack causes apathy, listlessness and depression, pallor, hypothermia, and thin, wrinkled skin. The eyes are sunken and muscles are wasted; wasting of temporal and masseter muscles is most noticeable in the early stages. The pulse may be slowed and the blood pressure lowered. Starvation oedema is dependent in type and not related solely to hypoproteinaemia. Body fat is lost. Milder degrees of this condition occur in the elderly, and it is often difficult to decide between a change due to age or a mild clinical abnormality.

Deficiency of fat

Lack of fat in the diet may lead to energy deficiency, but the most serious problem is lack of fat soluble vitamins, particularly vitamin D. Oily fish such as sardines are the richest dietary source of this hormone precursor.

Vitamin deficiencies

Vitamin A – Though some dietary surveys have shown a reduced intake of vitamin A, there is no real evidence to show related clinical problems. Vitamin A and carotenes are found in a wide variety of substances, dairy produce, fish oils, vegetables, and cereals.

Vitamin B₁ (thiamine) – Thiamine deficiency is occasionally seen in geriatric practice as either high output cardiac failure with considerable oedema and a dilated heart ("wet" beri-beri) or, very occasionally, the "dry" form with peripheral neuritis affecting the legs, burning paraesthesiae, cramps, weakness, and tender calves. The erythrocyte transketolase activity and the thiamine pyrophosphate effect tests are now used to assess thiamine state. Biochemical evidence of thiamine deficiency has been found in a large percentage of long stay patients,[6] but it has not been shown that repletion is of benefit to those without symptoms.[7]

Vitamin B₂ (riboflavine) and nicotinic acid – Deficiency of both these vitamins is shown by abnormalities of the mouth, tongue, and skin. Nicotinic acid deficiency causes cheilosis, angular stomatitis, and glossitis and may be complicated by diarrhoea, peripheral neuritis, and mental changes. The oral pathology may have other causes, such as iron deficiency or ill fitting dentures and the oral signs should be interpreted with caution. Nasolabial seborrhoea (enlarged, often red follicles near the sides of the nose with the follicles plugged with dry sebaceous material) occurs with riboflavine deficiency. The blood riboflavine concentration often does not correlate with the clinical state. The erythrocyte glutathione reductase activation coefficient test is now used to measure riboflavin state.

Folic acid – Nutritional folic acid deficiency is common among old people, though a macrocytic anaemia due to this is much less common. Serum folic acid concentrations below 2 μg/l probably indicate deficiency, but the red cell folate concentration is a better guide to tissue status.

Vitamin B₁₂ – A pure dietary cause for B₁₂ deficiency is rare, usually found only in vegans, but the incidence of atrophic gastritis and pernicious anaemia increases with age. Weight loss and anorexia may be features of pernicious anaemia. Diagnosis is not difficult when the disease presents classically. The diagnosis is most often made in the elderly by noting a raised mean cell volume on a blood report, by the haematologist seeing hypersegmented polymorphs, and/or a dimorphic blood picture denoting mixed microcytic and macrocytic anaemia. Neurological manifestations may occur without anaemia, and dementia due to low concentrations of vitamin B₁₂ in the cerebrospinal fluid and normal concentrations in the serum has been described.

Vitamin C – Scurvy may present with minimal signs. Royston's curls, hairs coiled on to the surface of the skin by a hyperkeratotic plaque, are more numerous over the anterior abdominal wall. Haemorrhage occurs around the hair follicle, and petechical haemorrhages occur, often first appearing on the ankles and feet. Patients with severe scurvy may have large spontaneous ecchymoses affecting muscles and skin, and haemarthroses. Subperiostial haemorrhages cause severe pain. Gingivitis can occur but not in the edentulous. Historical accounts of scurvy by sailors emphasise the severe lassitude and death following minor exertion. Scurvy now tends to affect those who cannot cook (widowers), those with bizarre diets, or those habituated to a gastric diet prescribed long ago. Patients in institutions are highly vulnerable; mass catering destroys vitamin C, so that not only may the basic diet be deficient but a plentiful supply of fresh fruit may not be available. The white cell ascorbic acid concentration is an indication of tissue status, but the vitamin C saturation test is a rare example of a truly therapeutic investigation. The recommended minimum daily amount of vitamin C required to maintain health is usually held to be 30 mg. The requirement for optimum benefit is, however, not known. Some hold it to be as high as 3000 mg/day. Vitamin C requirements increase with wound healing, and patients with bed sores, varicose ulcers, or large wounds may be given 1000 mg/day.

Vitamin D – A patient with severe osteomalacia is easy to diagnose. Backache, bone pains and tenderness, fractures, and a proximal myopathy with, perhaps, Chvostek's or Trousseau's signs are suggestive clinical findings. Demonstration of Looser's zones radiologically, low concentrations of serum calcium and phosphorus, and a high alkaline phosphatase activity help establish the diagnosis. A bone biopsy is confirmatory but often not essential. Calcidiol and calcitriol, the major circulating metabolites of vitamin D, can now be measured but the correlation with bone disease for an individual patient is not high. Studies of populations of elderly in homes and institutions, those who are housebound, and those with fractured neck of femur show low values of these metabolites, and a serum calcidiol concentration below 10 nmol/l indicates low vitamin D stores. These people also lack exposure to sunlight and dietary vitamin D. Malabsorption of cholecalciferol has been demonstrated in old people, and hepatic and renal hydroxylation are impaired with aging.[8] Patients with osteomalacia respond well to calcium and vitamin D. A major problem is whether supplementation prevents osteomalacia and fractures and improves muscle function in patients with low vitamin D stores who are asymptomatic. In spite of the lack of evidence to support supplementation it seems reasonable to ensure an adequate intake of calcium and exposure to unfiltered summer sunlight for old people. Solar irradiation is the most important source of vitamin D; dietary intake should only be necessary for those who cannot gain access to sunlight. The newer synthesised metabolites such as alphacalcidol are only necessary if renal disease is present. Usually calciferol in a dose of up to 0.25 mg (10 000 IU) a day will replenish vitamin D stores without risk of toxicity, though the serum calcium should be monitored. Solar exposure very rarely causes vitamin D toxicity.

Mineral deficiencies

Calcium – The normal intake of calcium is 800–1000 mg/day. The body is remarkably efficient at conserving calcium when the intake is low. Hypocalcaemia, with the development of tetany and cardiac arrest, can occur if vitamin D is given to a calcium deficient patient.

Iron – Iron deficiency anaemia is common in the elderly owing to gastrointestinal blood loss from a carcinoma, diverticulitis, hiatus hernia, or peptic ulcer or a low intake and poor absorption due to drugs or gut disease. The patient with iron deficiency anaemia due to occult gastrointestinal bleeding merits endoscopic and radiological investigation.

Potassium – An old person's diet often lacks potassium, and hypokalaemia is precipitated all too easily by diarrhoea or diuretic therapy. Combined thiazide potassium preparations may help prevent this, but supplementation with fruit or fruit juices should be advised.

Zinc – Zinc depletion delays wound healing and diuretics increase loss of this mineral. Zinc sulphate, 220 mg three times a day by mouth for two weeks, is often prescribed for patients with large bed sores or varicose ulcers.

Management of undernutrition

It is most important to identify the underlying cause of undernutrition and to search for occult disease causing anorexia or malabsorption. Modern endoscopic techniques and non-invasive investigations such as ultrasound, isotope scans, and computed tomography have greatly eased the problem of investigating frail old people. An accurate diagnosis is often more important for good management than for selecting treatment.

The patient may be helped by a supplementary pension, a home help, or meals on wheels. Rehousing, especially sheltered housing, may improve matters. An institution is a last resort, not without its own dangers.

Without doubt the best treatment is preventive, and good dietary advice should and does form part of preretirement education. During the initial phase of severe malnutrition high energy supplements containing vitamins and minerals are available which are very palatable. Parenteral feeding is sometimes indicated for emaciated or dysphagic patients. Narrow bore tubes for Clinifeed are easily tolerated for long periods, though the nutrient is very expensive. When malnutrition is less severe a normal diet should be supplemented with the specific minerals and vitamins. The number of pills should be kept to a minimum; the more there are, the less the compliance.

The patient who will not eat and visibly fades away is fortunately an infrequent problem. It can be difficult to decide how energetic the treatment should be, and an intubated patient struggling to die needs a humane approach. Adding life to years and not years to life should always be the guideline of treatment.[9]

[1] Exton-Smith AN, Stanton BR. *Report of an investigation into the dietary status of elderly women living alone.* London: King Edward's Fund for London, 1965.
[2] Berry WTC, Darke SJ. Nutrition of the elderly living at home. *Age Ageing* 1972; 1: 177–81.
[3] Davies L. Nutrition and malnutrition. In: Andrews J, Von Hahn HP, eds. *Geriatrics for everyday practice.* Basel: Skarger, 1981.
[4] Exton-Smith AN, Stanton BR. *A longitudinal study of the dietary of elderly women.* London: King Edward's Fund for London, 1970.
[5] MacLennan WJ. Nutrition of the elderly in continuing care. In: Caird FI, Grimley Evans J, eds. *Advanced geriatric medicine 3.* London: Pitman Medical, 1983.
[6] Brocklehurst JC, Griffiths LL, Taylor GF *et al.* The clinical features of chronic vitamin deficiency. *Gerontologia Clinica* 1968; 10: 309–20.
[7] Macleod RDM. Abnormal tongue appearances and vitamin status of the elderly – a double blind trial. *Age Ageing* 1972; 1: 99–102.
[8] Corless D. Vitamin D in the elderly. *J Clin Exp Gerontol* 1984; 6: in press.
[9] Lord Amulree. *Adding life to years.* London: Bannisdale Press, 1951.

Treatment of the "irremediable" elderly patient

BERNARD ISAACS

Here is a title as full of questions as a pomegranate is full of seeds. How does one treat the irremediable? If the irremediable is treated, is it irremediable? Is "to treat" less than "to remedy"? And why the contiguity of "irremediable" and "elderly"? Are all elderly irremediable? Are all irremediable elderly? These questions concern attitudes. They are important because attitudes rather than expertise determine the outcome of treatment.

Attitudes

There was a time, before I entered on that state of grace peculiar to the geriatrician, when the phrase "treatment of the irremediable elderly patient" would have concisely defined geriatrics for me. Later, when I began to work in geriatric medicine, I would have indignantly rebutted the implication that anyone or anything old was irremediable; for did we not profess our faith in the liturgical phrase: "an ill old person is ill because he is ill and not because he is old"? Now, after years of pragmatic practice of my art, I welcome the recognition that we geriatricians, and not we alone, devote much of our activities to the treatment of the irremediable. Few diseases at any age are cured; most whisper to the patient of their continuing presence, long after the ink is dry on the discharge letter. The treatment of the irremediable is both a worthy objective and an accurate description of much modern medicine.

Who are the "irremediable"?

First, who are they not? They are not, and must not be confounded with, the undiagnosed. They are not the confused, the incontinent, the senile. Confusion and incontinence are symptoms of impaired function of the nervous system and bladder. The words give no information on cause or cure. The term "senility" offends the geriatrician; it requires an effort of will even to write it. In my mind's eye I see the word garbed in a cloak of black with the blood of ill old people dripping from its lanky fingers. A melodramatic image perhaps; but how often has the attachment of this label to an ill old patient spelt the end of diagnostic and therapeutic endeavour and condemned him to a slow death by stewing in his own urine?

Every ill person of whatever age has a right to a diagnosis; and only when this has been established is it possible to talk about remediability or irremediability. "Senility" is not a diagnosis; it spells relegation for the patient and abdication by the doctor. I look forward to the day when the word "senility" will have disappeared from acceptable medical terminology, as the word "insanity" has done.

Irreversible disease

Many pathological processes which are common in old age are at present irreversible. These include neoplasm, atherosclerosis, and neuronal degeneration – one or more of which accompany most old people on their last long journey to the grave. It is among these sadly disabled people that the doctor seeks opportunities for effective intervention; and opportunities abound.

Treating the irremediable

A man of 69 was seen for the first time two months after the onset of a right hemiplegia, and after failure of a trial of rehabilitation. The patient was bedfast, there was no return of movement to the affected side, he had a catheter in his bladder, and he was unable to speak or to comprehend. He had been found picking faeces from his rectum and smearing them on his locker. He disturbed other patients by shouting. He had struck out at the nurses and given his wife a black eye.

First the wife was interviewed. Who was this man? What kind of person was he? He had been a good husband, a loving father, abstemious, a steady and conscientious worker, a keen amateur gardener, a fit man, proud of his good health and work record, inclined to disparage those less healthy than himself. What did she know of his illness? What did she say to him when she visited? She talked to him; sometimes, she thought, he understood her; sometimes he pushed her away and turned his head away from her. Once he lifted his hand to her, a thing he never did in his life. Did she ever cry? She had gone home and wept to herself every night since his illness began but hadn't told anyone. Did she think he was going to die? She didn't know, but sometimes she found herself half wishing that he would, and that made her feel wicked. Had she told this to anyone? Not a soul. Had anyone told her what was likely to happen to her husband? No one.

Next the patient was examined. His tongue was dry, his rectum packed with hard dry faeces. There was a pressure sore on his heel; his urine was infected; his haemoglobin level had dropped. He couldn't speak or understand language but he could pick up situational clues. He could sing "Tipperary" with the words matching the tune; he could count up to 10 if he was started off; he could correctly identify "bottle," "tumbler," "spectacles." He could build toy blocks one on top of the other. He could match dominoes. He had no movement in his arm or leg but he could sit up in bed with minimal support. Suddenly, out of this irremediable situation, all kinds of opportunities of effective intervention were appearing, like crocuses piercing the wintry soil.

The nurses began first. They put him on a fluid chart, gave him adequate nourishing drinks, talking to him as they did so, telling him what they were trying to do, encouraging him to take the cup and drink himself, trying to find out what he would like – orange juice, milk, tea, beer, perhaps even a glass of whisky. They found his pipe, his false teeth, his razor and comb. They emptied his bowel, they gave him fruit. They put him in the bath twice a day, gave him a support to take pressure off his painful heel. They spigoted his catheter, emptied his bladder every two or three hours for a day or two, then tried him without the catheter, carefully showing him how to use a bottle and ensuring that there was one where he could reach it on his left side. They sent for his clothes and shoes. They got him up, dressed, shaved, hair brushed, and showed him his image in the mirror. With the help of the physiotherapist they put him in a self propelled wheelchair and taught him how to use his good foot to drive himself about.

The physiotherapist mobilised his limbs and trunk, stood him up with support to give him the feel of the ground under his feet. The occupational therapist trained him to assist in his own dressing. The speech therapist discovered routes of communication by gesture and situational clues and taught the relatives and the nurses how to exploit these. The doctor treated the accompanying urinary infection and anaemia, relieved pain, ensured sleep, conferred with relatives and with the therapeutic team. In the end the patient did not fully "recover" – but he regained self respect and a limited degree of independence. He became much less demanding and frustrated. He was able to go on outings and could spend an occasional weekend at home. He took up indoor gardening and filled the dayroom with pot plants. We did not "cure"

146

him of his irremediable disease but we were privileged to watch the tide of his personality begin to flow again over the dry sand of his disability.

Principles

All this required the full geriatric team. In the more usual setting of the patient's home or a general hospital ward the same basic principles apply. These are:

(1) Listen carefully to the patient. He will tell you what needs to be done.

(2) Make yourself available to talk to relatives in privacy. They too have needs.

(3) Information is the fuel of opinion. So do not hesitate to investigate, but keep the investigation relevant to possible treatment.

(4) No form of treatment should be rejected dogmatically; always the benefits should be weighed against the hazards. To secure comfort in the last days of life, risks are justified.

Investigation and surgical treatment

The undiagnosed are often the unremedied; so no patient should be denied investigation. Evaluation of the haemoglobin, blood urea, electrolytes, and blood sugar is a minimum. A chest x ray film may show unsuspected cancer, tuberculosis, or osteomalacia. Sternal marrow examination is well tolerated and should not be withheld on grounds of age alone. Barium meals seldom lead to useful treatment. Barium enemas are more often helpful but may be frustrated by non-retention or by faecal accumulations. Urine cultures often yield organisms, but their eradication less often relieves symptoms.

Surgery and anaesthesia are well tolerated and should not be withheld if they offer hope of improvement in the quality of life. Postoperative rehabilitation may be very successful, and old people can learn to use colostomies or artificial limbs.

Relief of symptoms

Intractable pain is mercifully rare in the elderly. Its adequate control requires timely relief with non-narcotising doses of potent drugs, a technique which needs organisation, but which yields benefits by relieving the fear of having to endure pain.

Dyspnoea is more common and more difficult to control. Good posture is best obtained at home by nursing the patient in a chair.

Adequate diuresis is sometimes resisted, because the patient and his relatives become exhausted by frequent potting. A catheter should be used without hesitation. Oxygen usually causes more anxiety and tension than it relieves.

Anorexia is treated by indulgence. Favourite foods and beverages are prescribed; and a glass of whisky or sherry acquires a new and glorious flavour through having been prescribed by the doctor.

Treating dehydration is important since ill old people do not experience thirst. Their fluid intake should be charted, aiming at an intake of 1500 ml a day. If they have difficulty in swallowing they should use a straw or a child's feeding cup. Their fluids can be given in the form of jelly or liquidised foods.

Constipation is compounded by lack of roughage in the diet, lack of physical exercise, poor somatic muscle tone and evacuating power, inadequate opportunity, and fear of discomfort, quite apart from any autonomic dysfunction. The provision of a commode which the patient trusts and is prepared to use is as important as the prescription of the correct laxative or suppository. Regular enemas are required; regular rectal examinations are even more important.

Sleep disturbances send the doctor off on a prescription odyssey, sailing from drug to drug in an endeavour to secure sleep by night and wakefulness by day. From time to time one stops all drugs and starts again at the beginning with one aspirin at 9 pm – and sometimes this works. The hot milky drink may secure sleep at night, but the full bladder may alert early waking.

Psychological features

Doctors are often urged to allow old people to die with dignity. I find this very difficult to do since I associate dignity with black silk hats, the measured tread, the grave nod of the head – at very least with ambulation, continence, and mental clarity – features which are lacking as death approaches. Near the end of life some old people become undignified, remove their clothing in public, and revile their dear ones with obscenities. Others lose self control and become irritable, demanding, and selfish; refuse to be left alone; moan repetitively; ceaselessly ask for drinks; or demand to be taken to the lavatory, do nothing, then wet themselves. These anxiety symptoms are hard for relatives to bear; and many have confided to me that the last months of a loved parent's life were the worst they had ever experienced.

These situations test to the utmost the doctor's capacity to treat the irremediable. He must listen, sympathise, reassure, explain. The relatives require our ears and our time, but the doctor can also give practical help by arranging day hospital care or short term admission.

Conclusion

Much of medical work is concentrated on the final months or year of life. The curative role of the doctor is being attenuated, but equal or greater professional satisfaction can be found by the skilled and perceptive treatment of "the irremediable."

Anaemia in the elderly

J H THOMAS

Anaemia is always pathological and the clinical impression of its presence or absence often erroneous; it is not a concomitant of aging. The reported incidence has varied greatly. Pincherle and Shanks[1] found it in only 0.42% of 2000 business executives, 300 of whom were over 60 years. On the other hand, Parsons et al,[2] in a community survey, found an incidence of 7.2% in men and 11.1% in women in the age group 65–74 and in 20.8% and 23.3% respectively in those who were older. The Health Department's Nutritional Panel[3] gave a figure of 7.3%, which was about the same for men and women. The incidence among hospital admissions is about 30%.

The following groups of old people are particularly at risk of developing anaemia: those living alone, with mental deterioration, with apathy or depression, over 75 years of age, with diminished mobility, who have had gastric surgery, and who have been anaemic in the past.

Causes

Occult bleeding from the gastrointestinal tract is a frequent cause, but others – including insufficient intake of nutrients, diminished absorption, and general disease – are also important. Contributory factors, such as atrophic gastritis, chronic infection, carcinoma, renal disease, and the development of antibodies may also be present, and several factors may operate simultaneously.

Red cells from the marrow circulate for about 120 days and are then destroyed by the reticuloendothelial system, their iron and globin being reutilised. Derangement at any stage leads to anaemia.

Deficiency anaemia

The deficiency anaemias are of paramount importance and may be classified according to the deficient haemopoietic factor.

Iron deficiency anaemia

Iron deficiency anaemia is the most common type. Haemoglobin formation is diminished, resulting in hypochromia with a low mean corpuscular haemoglobin of 27 pg or less. The red cells are usually smaller than normal. There is sideropenia and reduction of iron saturation to below 16%, a level below 10% being pathognomonic.[4] Marrow smear and sections have a diminished iron content. Serum ferritin is low.

In iron deficiency anaemia due to blood loss the latter has usually occurred from the gastrointestinal tract, and occult blood testing of the stools is useful in every anaemic patient. When repeat tests are positive x ray investigation of the gastrointestinal tract is necessary, provided the bleeding is not due to such causes as thrombocytopenia or a raised blood urea. Microscopic examination of the urine should also be part of routine investigation.

Vitamin B_{12} deficiency anaemia

In vitamin B_{12} deficiency red cell formation is defective. Macrocytes appear in the peripheral blood, and the marrow becomes megaloblastic.

The serum B_{12} value is below 111 pg/ml and usually considerably so. (It is important to remember that if a bacillary method is used for estimating this level antibiotic therapy, particularly of ampicillin, should have been discontinued for at least three days as otherwise the low value may be false.) Nevertheless, a true low value can be obtained when the peripheral red cell is normal or hypochromic.

Findings in pernicious anaemia include achlorhydria and improvement in vitamin B_{12} absorption when it is combined with intrinsic factor. Gastric parietal cell antibodies (IgG) are present in 80% and intrinsic factor antibodies (IgA) in 50% of cases. The incidence is around seven per 1000, though it is higher in those with rheumatoid arthritis or hypothyroidism. There is a familial pattern.

Other reasons for vitamin B_{12} deficiency are partial gastrectomy, malnutrition, ileal malabsorption, and increased utilisation of the vitamin by proliferating organisms in jejunal or duodenal diverticula.

151

Folate deficiency

Folate deficiency may be due to malnutrition; malabsorption from jejunal disease; secondary to drugs, particularly those used in epilepsy; increased utilisation, as in myelofibrosis; or excess loss, as in exfoliative dermatitis. The full clinical picture should be evaluated before a certain diagnosis is made. Measurement of the faecal fat may be necessary, and also x ray examination of the small intestine. Its incidence increases with age, presumably owing to dietary difficulties.

In folate deficiency the fully developed blood picture is indistinguishable from that produced by vitamin B_{12} deficiency, as the two factors are interrelated. The serum folate value is below 2.5 ng/ml and the red cell value less than 140 ng/ml of packed red cells; but this latter measurement is a poor guide when there is associated vitamin B_{12} deficiency.

Other deficiencies

In vitamin C deficiency the cells are normocytic, though an occasional macrocyte may be seen. In deficiency of vitamin B_6 (pyridoxine) there is hypochromia with a low mean corpuscular haemoglobin concentration because the utilisation of iron by the red cells is impaired. When due to idiopathic derangement of its metabolism primary acquired sideroblastic anaemia results, but similar "ringed" sideroblasts may be seen with folate deficiency anaemia, with certain drug therapy, or with a carcinoma – particularly of the stomach.

Mixed deficiencies

Mixed deficiencies are common and are pinpointed when the various serum values are determined in all anaemic patients. The cells may be dimorphic or normocytic, but no appearance excludes the diagnosis.

Presentation

When anaemia is of rapid onset there is weakness, shortness of breath, and giddiness, but when it develops slowly, as it usually does, the symptoms are often ascribed to aging. Mental changes, angina pectoris, or heart failure may all be the presenting features, together with apathy, depression, or diminished mobility. The overall picture can be one of multiple lesions, with the anaemia being part of a wide spectrum of diseases.

In making the diagnosis a full history must be taken, paying special attention to the social environment, mental state, and mobility. Diet and mastication should be assessed, and also bowel action. Previous surgery or anaemia should be noted. The physical examination must be complete as no system can be neglected for a possible cause. The sequence followed in the investigations depends a great deal on the clinical features. Laboratory tests are necessary. It is helpful for the family doctor if the advice of a physician or pathologist is readily available together with an open door to the pathology department. The tests that are necessary are directed towards the clarification of formation, destruction, and loss of the red blood cells.

Treatment

Iron deficiency

About 200 mg of elemental iron are given daily between meals and the same dosage continued for at least three months after the haemoglobin has reached normal levels, to replenish the body stores. If intake is unreliable the calculated deficiency may be corrected by intramuscular therapy.

Vitamin B_{12} deficiency

One thousand micrograms is given weekly for four doses and then three monthly unless there is renal or hepatic disease, when the same dosage is given two monthly owing to increased body turnover.[5] The reticulocytosis should reach its highest level by the seventh day. If the cell count is one million the injections should give rise to a reticulocytosis of 40 % of the red cells while with one of three million the response should be 10 %. Hydroxocobalamin is preferable to cyanocobalamin, and lifelong injections are necessary in pernicious anaemia, in ileal malabsorption, and when dietary inadequacy cannot be corrected. Care is also necessary to ensure that iron or folate deficiency, or both, does not develop. Hypokalaemia has to be guarded against.

Folate deficiency

Five milligrams of folic acid three times a day are given until the blood count is satisfactory and then the dose is reduced to 5 mg daily. The body stores of vitamin B_{12} must be normal as otherwise neurological complications develop. When the diagnosis is in doubt a cover dose of 500 μg B_{12} should be given three monthly or the

153

vitamin B_{12} serum level should be confirmed as being normal every six months. Only when there is a continued cause for the deficiency, such as malabsorption or antiepileptic therapy, need long term treatment be given.

Blood transfusion

Whole blood is necessary when there is acute blood loss, but otherwise haematinic therapy usually suffices. Sometimes, however, packed red cells, 400 ml or thereabouts, repeated if necessary, may be life saving when the severity of the anaemia has caused heart failure, mental confusion, or extreme apathy. Patients with aplastic anaemia have to be transfused regularly, and the procedure is often necessary when urgent surgery is contemplated or when early radiological investigation of the gastrointestinal tract is essential.

Primary anaemia

Chronic lymphatic leukaemia increases steadily with age, but chronic myeloid leukaemia and acute leukaemia peak in the over 60 age group.[6,7] Treatment is justified despite the rapidity of onset and progress of the acute. On the other hand, "laboratory" leukaemia of the lymphatic type needs only correction of anaemia. Specific treatment is not necessary.

Secondary anaemia

General diseases, such as chronic infection, acute rheumatoid arthritis and carcinoma, can so alter the metabolism of iron that an iron deficiency type of anaemia appears when there is no true iron deficiency.

"Marrow" anaemia

Complete aplasia is unusual, but relative marrow failure is fairly common. There is mild normocytic normochromic anaemia with a poor marrow response. The cause has not been elucidated, though it is probably multifactorial. Infiltration with fibrous, myelomatous, or neoplastic tissue may result in a leucoerythroblastic picture, which is characterised by a leucocytosis and a mixture of immature red and white blood cells.

Haemolytic anaemia

The overt type of haemolytic anaemia, due to increased fragility of the red cells or damage by toxins, drugs, or antibodies, is less common than the latent variety. In this variant the red cell life is reduced, though not enough to produce anaemia if the marrow is functioning normally. Defects in both the peripheral cells and the bone marrow may be present in renal failure, liver dysfunction, carcinoma, and terminal disease.

Management

The advisability or otherwise of home management depends on the degree of illness, the extent and type of anaemia, the availability of the hospital service, and the social circumstances of the patient. Several questions arise: Is the anaemia due to a primary blood disorder, such as leukaemia? Is it secondary to malnutrition, malabsorption, blood loss, drug therapy, or general disease? Is it separate from the other abnormalities that may be present? Most of the answers are obtained by studying the haemoglobin level, the blood film, and the absolute values; by taking a careful history paying particular attention to food intake; and by carrying out a detailed physical examination, noting the presence or absence of adenopathy, splenomegaly, purpura, and the tell tale signs of malnutrition, chronic infection, or carcinoma. Occult blood testing of the stools is necessary, and if the anaemia is refractory or the cause obscure consideration is given to the possible presence of hypoplasia or haemolysis. The level of blood urea may supply the answer.

Whenever suitable the treatment should be at home, but the anaemia should never be dismissed as an incidental finding, of little or no consequence, because the underlying cause may be of vital significance. Ideally, the serum values of iron, vitamin B_{12}, and folate should be obtained despite the complexity of their interrelationship; but it is justifiable to give all three haematinics as an emergency when the patient is seriously ill – though future management is simplified if a blood sample is taken beforehand.

Prevention

Anaemia has a high morbidity, and therefore every effort should be made to reduce its incidence. Two methods are practicable. Firstly, primary prevention, by ensuring that all elderly people receive adequate quantities of protein and of haemopoietic factors in their daily diet – that is, 10-12 mg iron, 2-4 μg B_{12}, 100 μg folate,

50 mg vitamin C, and 2 mg pyridoxine. Ignorance, poverty, prejudice, apathy, and isolation are some of the resisting forces. The other method is secondary prevention – by detecting and treating the early case — (that is, when the haemoglobin level is around 11.6 g per 100 ml) and thereby preventing, or delaying, progression. Regular home visiting by doctors or nurses, or both, is essential, and special attention should be paid to those at risk.[6]

[1] Pincherle G, Shanks J. Value of the erythrocyte sedimentation rate as a screening test. *Br J Soc Prev Med* 1967; **21**: 40.

[2] Parsons PL, Withey JL, Kilpatrick GS. The prevalence of anaemia in the elderly. *Practitioner* 1965; **195**: 656–60.

[3] *A nutrition survey of the elderly*. London: HMSO, 1972: 57 (Reports on Health and Social Subjects No 3).

[4] Wintrobe MM. *Clinical haematology*. 6th ed. London: Kimpton, 1967: 597.

[5] Adams JF, Boddy K. The cobalamins. In: Arnstein HRV, Wrighton RJ, eds. *A Glaxo Symposium*. Edinburgh and London: Churchill Livingstone, 1971: 166.

[6] Thomas JH, Powell DEB. *Blood disorders in the elderly*. Bristol: Wright, 1971.

[7] Powell DEB. Incidence and distribution of ante leukaemia in one district general hospital area. *Lancet* 1971; ii: 350.

Diseases of the motor system

W J NICHOLSON

The Registrar General's statistical review of England and Wales reveals that 19% of all deaths in the over 65s were directly attributed to diseases of the nervous system. In addition, the 4% of all deaths in the same age group caused by diseases of the arteries must include a proportion in which the central nervous system was affected. Mortality figures reflect morbidity; every geriatric department contains more patients in this disease category than in any other. Though patients over 65 constitute only 14% of the total population, they occupy over one third of NHS beds. With an annual rise of 100000 in the over 65s the need must increase. The present figure of 514000 for the over 85s is likely to rise to 832000 by the year 2011. Standardised mortality rates continue to decline; the average length of hospital stay increases with age. These facts indicate that elderly patients with diseases of the central nervous system must make formidable demands on resources. The incidence of stroke rises dramatically with age. Patients with stroke occupy 17000 NHS beds in the UK (25% of all geriatric beds) and account for about 4·6% of all resources.

Disease of the pyramidal system

By far the commonest disease of the central nervous system is a stroke, ranging from disabling hemiplegia to a transient ischaemic cerebral episode with rapid recovery. A stroke with paralysis warranting admission to hospital is more common than acute appendicitis; a general practitioner with a list of 3000 will see five new strokes each year and will have a similar number of disabled stroke survivors on his list. The annual incidence of stroke is two per 1000 of the total population, which means 110000 new cases of stroke each year in England and Wales. Three quarters of all patients are over the age of 65. There are 130000 stroke survivors living at home in the UK, and 93000 of these are severely handicapped.[1]

The onset of a stroke due to cerebral thrombosis or embolism is usually first noticed after a period of sleep or rest. The patient may rise from bed to go to the lavatory and promptly fall because of weakness of the leg. Relatives may become alarmed because the patient is vacant and confused after an afternoon nap; when the doctor arrives the patient appears normal again. This latter episode is typical of transient ischaemic cerebral episodes, which may recur with frequency and may be helped, especially in men, by aspirin 100 mg on alternate days.

The patient with a major stroke has motor weakness of both the arm and leg; initially there is flaccid muscle tone with sluggish reflexes, but after a few days the tone increases and the jerks become brisk. The plantar response is extensor. The motor weakness is rarely equal in both arm and leg, one limb having more paresis than the other depending on the arterial territory affected most. Occlusion of the anterior cerebral artery results in maximum motor weakness in the contralateral leg; occlusion of the middle cerebral artery produces paralysis greatest in the contralateral arm and face, with dysphasia if the dominant hemisphere is affected.

The last three decades have seen a revolution in the management and rehabilitation of the patient with a stroke.[2] In the early weeks after a stroke mortality is 50%, aspiration pneumonia or pulmonary embolism being final complications. Of the survivors, half regain independence in daily living activities outside hospital. After the acute stage, in which life maintenance procedures are paramount and hypertension and cardiac arrythmias are controlled, the best rehabilitation results are obtained by admitting selected patients to special stroke units.[3] Here ancillary forces can be concentrated and patients' morale can be maintained by seeing the progress of recovery in others.

Most patients with uncomplicated hemiplegia spend two to three months retraining to stand and walk. Improvement in motor power can still be expected for up to eight months. Patients who progress to the point of social rehabilitation at home must be followed up for at least two years in the outpatient department or in day hospital. Careful neurological analysis of every patient pays great dividends in successful rehabilitation. For most, recovery is slow but persistent. Problems may arise with painful hemiplegic shoulder, spasticity, contractures, constipation, and depression. For those with delayed recovery it is imperative to identify the barriers to progress[4]; these include dysphasia, cortical sensory deficit, impaired muscle joint position senses, or an associated psychiatric disturbance. Discussion with the physiotherapist and occupational therapist on the reasons for delayed recovery is essential. Since a stroke is a family illness discharge must be planned over weeks ahead. It is prudent for the occupational therapist to visit the home and advise on what help is required in the way of supporting rail, ramp, or aids in the kitchen. Such planning relieves the anxiety of relatives and secures maximum cooperation. Each year 17% of stroke survivors die while 10% have a further stroke.

Pseudobulbar palsy

During recovery from a stroke a second cerebrovascular accident may occur on the opposite side. If both areas of vascular occlusion are in the region of the internal capsule then pseudobulbar palsy may result. Pseudobulbar palsy occurs in patients who are hypertensive and is characterised by emotional lability, a spastic tongue, brisk jaw jerk, and an upper motor neurone lesion in all four limbs; death may result from aspiration pneumonia. The emotional lability is distressing for patient and relatives but can be alleviated with imipramine[6] or amitriptyline.[7]

Brain stem ischaemia

Vascular insufficiency or occlusion in the posterior cerebral circulation results in one of the brain stem syndromes. Here the patient is prostrated with severe giddiness, double vision, vomiting, and ataxia. On examination there is nystagmus, intention tremor in the ipsilateral limbs, and numbness in the ipsilateral face and contralateral side of the body. Ipsilateral involvement of a cranial nerve may be present. Despite the alarming onset the prognosis is good.

Motor neurone disease

As in younger people, motor neurone disease is characterised by weakness and wasting in all four limbs, fasciculation being greatest in the limb girdles; all limb reflexes are brisk, the plantars are extensor, and there is no sphincter disturbance. Prognosis for survival is more favourable than in younger people. Even with bulbar involvement there is a relatively better prognosis.[8]

Disease of the extrapyramidal system

In 1817 an east London general practitioner, Dr James Parkinson, published *An Essay on the Shaking Palsy*, which gave a lucid description of the clinical manifestation of disease of the

159

extrapyramidal system. Every general practice contains several patients with parkinsonism – who are easily remembered because of both their appearance and their need for repeat prescriptions. Parkinsonism or paralysis agitans is due to disease of the basal ganglia. Primary degeneration of unknown aetiology is the commonest cause, with degeneration secondary to vascular disease or to encephalitis lethargica being much less common. Drugs often cause parkinsonism, the chief offenders being methyldopa, reserpine, chlorpromazine, and the phenothiazines; haloperidol is notable for rapidly producing parkinsonian features. Parkinsonism caused by drugs is dose dependent. Clinically parkinsonism is recognised at a glance, from the fixed, expressionless gaze, infrequent blinking, and festinating walk in small steps with bent attitude. Half the patients exhibit the coarse compound tremor which may affect any or all of the limbs as well as the jaw. The tremor is present at rest but disappears with sleep and with voluntary movement; anxiety worsens the tremor. The limb reflexes are normal. The post-encephalitic type of parkinsonism, with seborrhoeic skin, drooling saliva, and oculogyric crisis, is rarely seen because there are now few survivors of the 1920 epidemic.

Treatment

The introduction of levodopa represented a major advance in therapeutics.[9] Unfortunately, not all patients are suitable for this treatment. It is a good working rule that to benefit a patient must be clear in the head. All levodopa preparations, even when initially successful, seem to show a decline in efficacy after two years,[9] with problems such as dyskinesias, the "on off" phenomenon, and freezing episodes.

In assessing the parkinsonian patient for initiation of therapy it is prudent to be influenced by the patient's disability. Before rushing into levodopa therapy it is worth while trying the older therapies such as orphenadrine or procyclidine together with physiotherapy. The earlier levodopa treatment starts the earlier will side effects appear. If increasing disability demands levodopa then the early side effects of postural hypotension, cardiac arrythmias, and confusion must be expected during the build up period. Once stabilised on a plateau dose of levodopa most patients do well for several years.

With the onset of diminishing levodopa efficacy bromocriptine can be started; the dose of bromocriptine should be gradually increased as that of levodopa is decreased.[10] Like levodopa bromocriptine may have troublesome side effects, such as postural hypotension and dyskinesias.

Hemiballismus

A vascular lesion of the subthalamic nucleus results in sudden onset of violent choreic movement in the contralateral half of the body. The violence of the movements rapidly exhausts the patient, and involvement of the pharyngeal muscles may result in aspiration pneumonia. Tetrabenzine is effective in relieving the movements, but the movements can be abolished with stereotaxic surgery.

Lower motor neurone lesion

Polyneuropathy represents the commonest lower motor neurone lesion of old age and is characterised by bilateral flaccid muscle weakness maximum in the distal limb muscles, always worse in the legs. There may also be sensory loss of the stocking and glove type. Most cases of peripheral neuropathy are mixed motor and sensory. Asymmetry is unusual in either the motor or the sensory component.

The clinical signs are weakness, sluggish or absent reflexes, wasting of the muscles, and tenderness of the muscles and soles of the feet; tenderness is a prominent feature of alcoholic neuropathy but may occur in the acute stage of any neuropathy. The sensory loss usually affects all modalities. Plantar responses are flexor or absent.

Diabetes mellitus is the most likely cause of a polyneuropathy in any old person. Routine urine testing cannot rule out the diagnosis, nor can one estimation of the blood sugar concentration. A glucose tolerance test should be performed in all cases when both urine tests and blood sugar concentrations are inconclusive. Most elderly diabetics are obese, and management of the polyneuropathy aims at arresting its progress by good diabetic control, preferably by diet supplemented if required by a sulphonylurea or a diguanide preparation. Diabetic peripheral neuropathy may be purely sensory and may affect only muscle joint and vibration sensations – hence the description of this condition as "diabetic pseudotabes." These patients may develop perforating ulcers in the feet and, with vascular impairment, great care must be taken in chiropody.

Polyneuropathy may be the presenting manifestation of a carcinoma, especially carcinoma of the bronchus, occurring long before the primary neoplasm is obvious. Herpes zoster, even a mild and limited infection, may be complicated by polyneuropathy.

Deficiency of vitamin B_{12} either in addisonian pernicious anaemia or in a malabsorption syndrome may result in polyneuropathy, but this may be associated with posterior column signs to cause subacute combined degeneration. Systemic therapy with vitamin

B_{12} will reverse the lesion in the lower motor neurone but will only arrest the lesion in the posterior column.

Alcoholism is a problem in the elderly, especially among women, who tend to drink alone at home. As well as peripheral neuropathy these patients may develop a gross memory defect or become confused; hence Korsakoff's psychosis may be diagnosed as senile dementia. Even though there is no scientific proof of its worth, it is traditional to give vitamin concentrates during a period of alcoholic withdrawal.

Gold, sulphonamides, nitrofurantoin, and isoniazid may all cause polyneuropathy. With polyneuropathy of any cause patients will become disabled and unable to walk. While the primary cause is being treated ambulation must be maintained or regained with physiotherapy.

1 Harris AI, Cox E, Smith CRW. *Handicapped and impaired in Great Britain. Part 1*. London: HMSO, 1971.
2 Adams GF. *Gerontologia Clinica* 1967; **9**: 285.
3 Royal College of Physicians of London. Geriatric Committee. Working Group on Strokes. *Report*. London: Royal College of Physicians of London, 1974.
4 Adams GF, Hurwitz LJ. Mental barriers to recovery from strokes. *Lancet* 1963; ii: 533–6.
5 Hurwitz LJ. Management of major strokes. *Br Med J* 1969; iii: 699–702.
6 Lawson IR, MacLeod RDM. The use of imipramine and other psychotropic drugs in organic emotionalism. *Br J Psych* 1969; **115**: 281–5.
7 Hamilton LD. *Clinical Medicine* 1966; **73**: 49.
8 Hodkinson HM. *Age Ageing* 1972; **1**: 182.
9 Marsden CD, Parkes JD. *Lancet* 1977; i: 345–9.
10 Anonymous. Levodopa: long term impact on Parkinson's disease [Editorial]. *Br Med J* 1981; **282**: 417–8.

Disturbances of the special senses and other functions

W J NICHOLSON

Sensory deprivation is known to be a powerful weapon in causing perceptual disturbances.[1] Maintenance of contact with reality demands stimulation from the environment,[2] and hence it is not surprising that old people who are deaf or blind, or both, appear to be confused – the links of communication to a sensorium with diminishing reserve have been severed. Social isolation and loss of independence are associated with loss of the special senses. These are compelling reasons for ensuring that every old person can see and hear to his or her maximum capacity.

Impairment of hearing is often made worse by hard plugs of wax; removal by syringing after several days' softening is a simple procedure. If deafness persists after removing the wax it is most likely to be due to either middle ear deafness or nerve deafness. A vibrating tuning fork is applied to the vertex of the skull in the midline, and the patient is asked (in writing if necessary) to indicate whether she hears the sound in the midline or in either ear (Weber's test); in middle ear deafness the sound is localised in the affected ear but in nerve deafness it is localised in the normal ear. In Rinne's test the vibrating tuning fork is applied to the mastoid process, the ipsilateral ear being closed. The patient is asked to indicate when the sound ceases, and the vibrating tuning fork is then placed over the ipsilateral ear. In middle ear deafness nothing can be heard, but in nerve deafness the sound can still be heard. Patients with middle ear deafness have conductive hearing loss and benefit from a bone conduction hearing aid. Damaged structures in the cochlea and auditory nerve result in sensorineural deafness, in which conventional hearing aids are of little value. Patients with total bilateral hearing loss constitute only 2% of those with sensorineural deafness. Most of the sensorineural deaf have some residual hearing but because of frequency loss of "ski slope" distribution find little help from an amplifying hearing aid. The few patients suitable for insertion of single channel implant prosthesis are helped because the conduction provided is an aid to lip reading.[3] It is imperative when conversing with an old patient always to talk directly into the face, preferably at eye level. Many deaf patients get by with clever lip reading. Otosclerosis is the commonest cause of middle ear deafness; rarer causes are Menière's disease, acute labyrinthitis, trauma, and treatment with streptomycin or ethacrynic acid. β Blockers can cause reversible hearing impairment of mixed type with an air bone gap sparing the middle ear.[4] If the ipsilateral corneal reflex is absent in the deaf patient then investigation for acoustic neuroma must be made.[5]

There are over 120000 registered blind people in Britain, 3·4% of whom have no perception of light. The association of diabetes mellitus and blindness is a compelling reason always to aim for good blood sugar concentrations to avoid diabetic retinopathy. Sudden loss of vision in either eye demands urgent specialist attention. Acute glaucoma, arteritis, internal carotid artery occlusion, and detached retina all cause sudden deterioration in vision and are treatable. A detached retina is recognised when a well demarcated area of the retina is seen moving like a sail with a well defined margin; often there is associated haemorrhage into the vitreous. A pale optic disc with unfilled blood vessels is seen in carotid occlusion. A profuse haemorrhagic area indicates a venous thrombosis – usually limited to one venous segment. Primary optic atrophy is recognised by the appearance of a well defined pale disc with the attenuation of all blood vessels; treatment of the cause such as syphilis can arrest the deterioration in vision. Unilateral or asymmetrical primary optic atrophy may result from a pituitary tumour or a sphenoidal wing meningioma. Macular degeneration produces blindness on a spot in the centre of the page and therefore is less hazardous than the tunnel vision of chronic glaucoma, which leads to bumping into or falling over objects. Paget's disease of the skull may compress optic nerves, with blindness, and the eighth nerves, with deafness. Elderly people may have primary optic atrophy from toxic exposure in earlier life such as tobacco, quinine, methyl alcohol, or inorganic arsenic about which nothing can be done. A hemianopia is invariably associated with a hemiplegia or some other evidence of a stroke.

Headache

Headache is not a feature of hypertension or space occupying lesions in the elderly.

The headache of temporal arteritis represents an emergency because of the danger of sudden blindness due to occlusion of the ophthalmic branch of the internal carotid artery.[6] The patient with temporal arteritis may be vaguely unwell with limb pains and pyrexia; alternatively, the condition may present with sudden headache and vomiting. The erythrocyte sedimentation rate is always raised. Examination of the temporal or occipital arteries will reveal a tender swollen artery which does not pulsate. The pathological process is one of gradual arterial occlusion and therefore warrants immediate treatment with steroids (60 mg prednisolone daily). To avoid the dangers of long term steroid treatment the affected artery should undergo biopsy because this minor operation seems to result in remission of the arteritis.

Cervical spondylosis is a common cause of occipital headache. Glaucoma may present with headache, vomiting, and photophobia; the increased intraoccular tension differentiates it from subarachnoid haemorrhage and meningitis. Headache due to arthritis of the temperomandibular joint is episodic and always worse at meal times. Sinusitis produces a headache which builds up to maximum intensity in the early afternoon and subsides towards evening; often there is an associated upper respiratory infection. Tension headache is common and is recognised by the patient's description of it being "like a weight on top" or "a band around the head"; headache associated with depression is recognised from other indicators in the symptoms.

Facial pain

Trigeminal neuralgia or tic douloureux has its highest incidence in elderly women, being characterised by a paroxysmal sharp pain in the second or third division of the trigeminal nerve. The pain begins suddenly and usually lasts about 30 seconds; eating, talking, touching the face, or a cold wind may precipitate an attack. Spasm of the affected side of the face may occur, with closing of the eye and lachrymation. There are no abnormal physical signs between attacks. The waxing and waning nature of this affliction is seen in the middle aged but it wanes less often in the old patient, who may develop a depressive illness. Dental malocclusion or temperomanibular dysfunction, especially in adentulous patients, may precipitate attacks of trigeminal neuralgia and should be treated.[7]

The introduction of carbamazepine has changed the management of trigeminal neuralgia; rarely is alcohol injection or surgical resection of the trigeminal ganglion required. The side effects of giddiness and drowsiness make it imperative to introduce carbamazepine gradually, from 100 mg once daily to a maximum dosage of 200 mg thrice daily. This drug is an anticonvulsant with the usual toxic effects of agranulocytosis and a plastic anaemia. If intolerance develops phenytoin 100 mg twice daily can be given together with a tetracyclic antidepressant or chlorpromazine.

Herpes zoster

Herpes zoster, or shingles, has its highest incidence in older patients. It is an acute virus infection affecting the first sensory neurone with a papulovesicular eruption in the corresponding dermatome. A few days of pain in the dermatome often precede the appearance of the segmental rash. Dusting powder and dry dressings of the eruption are usually all that is necessary, but if there is secondary infection then systemic rather than local antibiotic treatment is indicated. Zoster may affect the ophthalmic division of the fifth cranial nerve, with corneal lesions and the risk of optic neuritis; when the sight is in jeopardy systemic steroid treatment is needed. Rarely zoster affects the geniculate ganglion, with pain in the ear, lower motor neurone facial paralysis, giddiness, deafness, and loss of taste in the anterior two thirds of the tongue (Ramsay Hunt's syndrome). Most patients with herpes zoster recover without complications, the rash subsiding after seven days; however, a few develop postherpetic neuralgia, with intractable pain associated with depression. Many therapies have been tried for this condition but none seem any more effective than simple analgesics.

Vertigo

Vertigo can be a crippling malady. The commonest cause is postural hypotension. Normally the blood pressure remains constant irrespective of the posture; this independence of posture is maintained by baroreceptor reflexes operating from the aorta and the carotid sinuses. In old age the postural change requires a longer time for a baroreceptor adjustment, especially when cerebrovascular disease is present[8]; hence rapid standing up can cause momentary dizziness. Old people should get out of bed in three stages[9]: they should first sit up, then dangle their legs over the side of the bed, and finally stand up. That an elderly person who feels giddy has postural hypotension can easily be confirmed by recording the blood pressure lying down, sitting, and standing. Only one reading, taken lying down, can be deceptive. Postural hypotension is a manifestation of various diseases which interrupt or slow down the baroreceptor efferent pathway and commonly it is seen in patients who are recovering from an illness with imposed immobility – for example, a stroke or congestive cardiac failure. In these instances gradual re-education of the baroreceptor reflexes occurs with increasing mobility.

Autonomic neuropathy, as in diabetes mellitus, tabes dorsalis, or acute infective polyneuropathy, is a rare cause of postural hypotension. Drugs often cause troublesome postural hypotension; not surprisingly, adrenergic blockers do so, but many other therapeutic agents also lower the blood pressure as a side effect – for example, diuretics, barbiturates, phenothiazines, the tricyclic antidepressants, and the antiparkinsonian drugs.

Giddiness associated with neck movement is rarely a symptom in patients with cervical spondylosis; the atheromatous vertebral arteries are further narrowed by cervical osteophytes with added ischaemia on neck movement. Other evidence of cervical spondylosis, such as wasting of the arm muscles or a spastic paraparesis, will be present.[10] A cervical collar may help the giddiness.

Menière's disease

Menière's disease represents acute loss of vestibular function and may present for the first time in old age. The patient may have felt deaf for some time but then suddenly experiences tinnitus in one ear associated with a violent rotary sensation, vomiting, profuse sweating, and prostration. There is rotatory nystagmus maximum to the side of the affected ear and an intention tremor on the finger-nose test. Chlorpromazine 50 mg intramuscularly is useful in the acute attack to control vomiting but diuretic therapy to reduce the swollen endolymphatic system is disappointing. When increasing tinnitus heralds another episode dramamine or torecan can be given. With increasing disability a unilateral labyrinthectomy may be necessary, sacrificing hearing for balance.

Drop attacks

Old people often fall, but when a drop attack is the cause there is a history of the patient falling without warning, not losing consciousness, and not having amnesia.[11] A patient may be standing or walking when the episode occurs; the patient rises quickly again; and there are no abnormal physical signs in the legs. Such attacks appear related to sudden failure of extensor tone in the legs. There is no known treatment, but drop attacks wax and wane in frequency and often remit completely. Variable heart block, a Stokes Adams attack, basilar artery insufficiency, and epilepsy are the main differential diagnoses.

Subdural haematoma

The highest incidence of subdural haematoma is in the elderly and in infants, with males predominating. Trauma is the commonest cause, but a history of this is often unobtainable, and when a good history is obtained the trauma may have been minimal. There is an association with alcoholism. The diagnosis is easy if the symptoms immediately follow an injury, but this is rarely the case; more often there is an insidious onset weeks or months after the injury with fluctuating headache, drowsiness, and confusion.[12] Focal cerebral symptoms are unusual but when present give a clinical picture resembling a stroke. Subdural haematoma is frequently bilateral. Electroencephalography is a disappointing test. The isotope scan may be more informative than the computed tomogram. Angiography shows displacement of the cerebral arteries away from the inner table of the skull.

Epilepsy

About half the seizures that occur in the elderly are associated with cerebrovascular disease, 15 % are caused by tumour, while the remainder are secondary to extracerebral causes. The onset usually follows a stroke, the seizure is grand mal in type, and Jacksonian episodes are infrequent. A history of a recent stroke and the association of an upper motor neurone lesion in one or more limbs will be associated evidence. The fits can be controlled with primidone or phenytoin. Uraemia, hypoglycamia, and variable heart block may all provoke epileptiform seizures. In those patients with late onset epilepsy for which there is no obvious cause it is always a difficult problem to balance the points for and against a full neurological investigation; one should be influenced by the patient's biological rather than chronological age. Postictal confusion and paralysis (Todd's paralysis) both last longer in the older patient and may cause diagnostic problems if a history of a fit is not known.

The dementias

There is wide individual variation in intellectual impairment in old age. Over the age of 80 the incidence of dementia is 20 %. Acute confusion occuring on change of environment often unmasks the early dementing process. For treatment and management it is mandatory to find the aetiology of the dementia. Dementia secondary to vascular change is associated with lateralising neurological signs such as a hemiplegia or bilateral extensor plantar responses. Other evidence of vascular disease is often found – for example, coronary artery disease, peripheral vascular disease, or hypertension. Senile dementia of the Alzheimer type is not associated with neurological signs or vascular change. Prognostically the distinction is important. Patients with arteriosclerotic dementia are likely to survive longer, with waxing and waning, but those with Alzheimer's dementia have an unremitting downhill course and rarely survive more than two years after the diagnosis is made. Evidence suggests that Alzheimer's dementia has a genetic basis, but few patients who carry the gene survive to the age when the effects are obvious.[13] A treatable cause of dementia is normal pressure hydrocephalus. Dementia associated with abnormalities of gait (especially marche aux petits pas) makes one suspect this lesion. The aetiology and incidence are undetermined, but these patients may improve after shunting of the ventricular cerebrospinal fluid into the venous system.[14,15]

Conclusion

Maintenance of cerebration, ambulation, sight, and hearing are essential for the quality of life and for an independent existence. The essentials depend more on the integrity of the central nervous system than on any other system.

[1] Brown JAC. *Techniques of persuasion*. Harmondsworth; Penguin Books, 1973: 246.

[2] Slade PD. *Br J Hosp Med* 1984; **32**: 256.

[3] Velmans ML. New ears for old: auditory implants and frequency transposing hearing aids. *J R Coll Physicians Lon* 1982; **16**: 83.

[4] Fält R, Liedholm H, Aursnes J. β Blockers and loss of hearing. *Br Med J* 1984; **289**: 1490.

[5] Parker HL. Tumours of nervus acusticus: signs of involvement of fifth cranial nerve. *Arch Neurol Psych* 1928; **20**: 309.

[6] Allison RS. *The senile brain*. London: Arnold, 1963: 45.

[7] Blairgas GDS. Trigeminal neuralgia and dental malocclusion. *Br Med J* 1973; iv: 38.

[8] Gross M. The effect of posture on subjects with cerebrovascular disease. *Quart J Med* 1970; **39**: 485.

[9] Anderson WF. *Practical management of the elderly*. Oxford: Blackwell, 1967: 96.

[10] Brain WR, Northfield DWC, Wilkinson M. Neurological manifestations of cervical spondylosis. *Brain* 1952; **75**: 187.

[11] Sheldon JH. On the natural history of falls in old age. *Br Med J* 1960; ii: 1685.

[12] McKissock W, Richardson A, Bloom WH. Subdural haematoma: a review of 389 cases. *Lancet* 1960; i: 1365.

[13] Isaacs B. *Introduction to geriatrics*. London: Balliere, Tindall and Cassell, 1965: 108.

[14] Anonymous. Dementia and normal pressure hydrocephalus. *Lancet* 1970; ii: 1074.

[15] Anonymous. Normal pressure hydrocephalus and psychiatric disorders. *Br Med J* 1973; ii: 260.

Geriatric orthopaedics

MICHAEL DEVAS

In good health the aged have to face many problems in any society; to them illness comes as a catastrophe which can take away their independence. The life expectancy of a young adult is increasing, but never more so than in the West. This is not the only cause of increased problems, because certain conditions, such as fractures near the hip, show an absolute increase in incidence over and above that of the increase in the elderly population. Because of this geriatric orthopaedics is a most important and stimulating subject, with many rewards in achieving independence for patients. To treat the elderly properly makes great demands on both medical and surgical skills and requires enthusiastic team work from all those concerned if the essential objective of treatment – to restore a proper quality of life – is to be achieved.

The principles of geriatric medicine and surgery are the same as at any other age but they have to be applied with the utmost vigour from the moment of admission to the ultimate discharge from outpatients. The circumstances in which the patient lives, financial problems, the surgical condition, concomitant medical afflictions, how rehabilitation and the social services can best be used, nursing care, and, most important, the morale of the patient all have to be carefully considered. It must be remembered that in the elderly loss of function means loss of independence.

The most important physical sign in geriatric orthopaedics is to see the patient walk. The next most important is to see that the patient can undertake the ordinary activities of daily living. Hence all treatment must be aimed at restoring both as quickly as possible. An old person invariably has many other ailments besides that which caused the admission to hospital, especially when the admission is caused by a fracture. Treatment is therefore best managed by a team based on a special geriatric orthopaedic unit, to which the more enfeebled patient may be transferred as soon as possible after operation.

There are two main divisions of surgical treatment: the emergency repair of a fracture and the elective orthopaedic operation. In each, however, the aim of returning the patient to a satisfactory quality of life as soon as possible is the same.

In geriatric orthopaedics, however, it has become apparent that the shorter the time the patient spends in hospital the better the outcome. A fracture near the hip, for example, is totally incapacitating. If treatment is not started very quickly and total care instituted on admission the quality of life will suffer. Bed rest in the elderly is bad mainly because it hinders the restoration of normal activities. Prolonged decubitus adds to the osteoporotic problems; mental blurring of the normal day to day activities is apparent; and there are many other contraindications, such as respiratory, genitourinary, and other intercurrent infections. In the very elderly in particular postural hypertension can become a considerable problem and if left unrecognised may prevent the return to normal function.

For these reasons the best surgical procedure for an old patient is one that allows the patient to start walking as soon as she or he wakes from the anaesthetic. In the treatment of fractures no operation should be done that leaves the patient in bed, suffering not only from the effects of the broken bone but also from those of the operation. The operation is well tolerated in the elderly but it must be considered to be merely an incident in the general rehabilitation of the patient.

Fractures near the hip

A fracture near the hip is the commonest emergency and one which can cause serious social, medical, and surgical difficulties. A fractured hip exemplifies the problems of management, treatment, and rehabilitation in all geriatric orthopaedic conditions.

An old person who fractures the hip at home will normally be seen by her own doctor, who can start treatment immediately. First he should make the patient comfortable where she lies, not causing pain by lifting her to a couch or chair but padding the back, heels, and sacral area. Next, and most important, he should reassure the patient and tell her that under normal circumstances her stay in hospital will be short, perhaps a week, and that after that she will be transferred to nursing home type accommodation for a short period before coming home. In this way the patient knows before going into hospital that treatment will be quick and that the broken hip will soon be mended. Once the patient has understood this, the doctor must then, and this is equally important, reassure relatives and neighbours with the same advice.

The patient is taken to hospital in an ambulance, which should have a thick foam mattress already in place on the stretcher. Pressure sores often start even before the patient is on a stretcher from lying on a hard floor for an hour or so before help arrives. In hospital the patient should remain on the thick foam mattress on the hospital trolley, from which she should not be moved until she has finally been put into her own bed. Unnecessary movement causing pain must be avoided because the more the patient is moved with a painful fracture the worse is the shock that might be sustained.

Radiographs should be taken of the affected part and of the lung fields. Routine blood tests should be done, heart failure and diabetes excluded, and, if there is much pain, skin traction applied to the affected limb, but using foam traction rather than adhesive. Except for the few patients with unstable diabetes and untreated heart failure, the patient is prepared for operation, which should be done within 24 hours. Those with diabetes or heart failure may have to wait for a few hours, but even they should not normally have their operation delayed beyond 24 hours. Before operation the dehydrated patient should be given fluids intravenously, and at operation blood should be given freely. Packed cells are of great value to avoid overloading the circulation in very anaemic patients. An antibiotic is given routinely to cover the operation, but streptomycin should not be used in the elderly.

There are no statistics available on whether it is better to operate on an old person's hip as soon as possible or wait for the next operating list, but experience suggests that waiting for the next list is best. Normally a patient is not ready for theatre until late at night and, without special night teams, the work of the orthopaedic department in a normal sized hospital is disrupted, with a possible lowering of technical standards. Nevertheless, there is never an indication, because of the age of the patient or her general feebleness, to delay operation, for this merely allows the patient to run into all those problems caused by bed rest, particularly when the bed rest is associated with pain on movement.

The elderly patient who is allowed to lie in hospital in pain and discomfort brings opprobrium to the department in whose bed she lies when the only contraindication to operation is age or decrepitude. That old people die is accepted by patients, but there is a tendency among some surgeons not to worry about death before operation, however miserable and unhappy it may be, but to take more than necessary steps to try to preserve life afterwards. The surgeon who operates on all old people as they come will have the greater gratitude extended to him even if his mortality rate appears high.

Furthermore, patients with a short life expectancy should still have the benefit of having their fracture mended so that their last days, even if in hospital, may at least be comfortable. A fracture at the hip causes pain, particularly when a bedpan is used, so, however ill the patient, the operation should not be shirked.

Anaesthesia

Apart from heart failure and diabetes, there are rarely any contraindications to early anaesthesia. Indeed, the earlier it is given the better the outlook for the patient because of the ability to clear out the lungs during the anaesthetic and to ventilate them properly throughout.

If a general anaesthetic is to be used oxygen must be given freely throughout. There is a considerable body of opinion that believes that lack of oxygen for any period increases the possibility of confusion after the operation and this, of course, applies to any period of anoxia during recovery. Therefore, all old people must be watched with particular care. In old age the pharyngeal muscles lose tone, thereby making airway obstruction relatively easy to occur in the period after operation.

Sucking out the bronchial tree and giving blood to the normally anaemic old person are probably the most important features of a general anaesthetic.

Spinal anaesthesia is gaining favour, but the procedure, whether intrathecal or epidural, is uncomfortable because the patient has to be turned and this may cause pain however great the care. As yet there is little indication of which gives the better results.

Bladder care

Women should undergo catheterisation before operation, and the catheter should be left in place for 48 hours, when it can usually be removed. Men must also be catheterised if there is any suspicion of an enlarged prostate or other urinary problem. If after removal of the catheter there is difficulty in micturition the catheter should be replaced for a few days and again withdrawn. This usually works but if it does not cystoscopy is needed, and often simple bladder neck resection in men restores normality.

Choice of operation

There are two main types of broken hip: the fractured neck of femur and the trochanteric fracture. The fractured neck of femur is probably still best treated by immediate replacement with a hemiarthroplasty and the trochanteric fracture by some form of pin and plate fixation. Both forms of treatment have problems, however. With the advancing age of the patient and the increased risk of osteoporosis it is not possible to guarantee that any internal fixation device will not cut out of the neck of the femur when the patient starts to walk. As the object of the operation is to enable the patient to walk immediately the complication has to be accepted, but the patients should be watched carefully for this complication.

The normal form of replacement for a fractured neck of femur has been the Thompson or Austin Moore prosthesis, but both these have been shown to produce an unacceptable rate of acetabular erosion after operation, which implies that the head of the prosthesis wears into the acetabulum and may penetrate upwards to such a degree that it enters the pelvis. The morbidity occasioned by this means that at least half of all patients with this erosion of the acetabulum may require total hip replacements. To prevent this complication, however, a new bipolar prosthesis (the Hastings hip, manufactured by Charles Thackray, Leeds) has been produced in which the head articulates on a smaller inner head. Early results with this prosthesis are good, and acetabular erosion appears to all intents to have been eliminated. Furthermore, the procedure is simple, and the new head is easier to fit than the Thompson or Austin Moore prosthesis. It also provides a much more accurate method of restoring the normal anatomical configuration of the hip, which means that the patient, having no shortening and an accurately sized new femoral head replacement, has more confidence in walking afterwards.

The principle of the Hastings hip is that the acetabulum is measured extremely accurately by means of a special sizer: its diameter can be assessed to within 0·5 mm. A suitable outer head, or cup, of the correct diameter is then chosen, but the stem remains the same for each size of cup. Furthermore, because of the design, with each step the patient takes the outer head moves to align itself with the thrust of weight bearing through the hip, and movement therefore, occurs not only at the inner interprosthetic articulation but also between the prosthesis and the acetabulum.

Operation and after care

It is not necessary to go into the technical details of the various operations other than to emphasise that bedsores can occur even on a theatre table; that the technique must be painstaking but gentle; that speed is important but accuracy should not be sacrificed to it; and that careful haemostasis is vital. Antibiotic powder should be sprinkled into the wound.

The wound is closed in layers with one or two suction drains.

An air permeable adhesive dressing covers the incision. The patient will walk the next day whether the hip has been treated by internal fixation or by a hemiorthoplasty. Done properly, the operation has few complications other than those mentioned above, which occur late. Dislocation of the prosthesis is very rare.

A lateral approach should always be used in approaching the fractured hip in the elderly. It is not near the perineum, so incontinence does not present a risk of contamination to the wound and, not being posterior, the approach allows the patient to lie or sit comfortably. With the anterior approach, flexion of the hip causes movement of the sutured skin edges and often the inguinal crease has some intertrigo.

After the operation analgesics should be given to control pain adequately. The antibiotic started before the operation should be continued for five days and longer if there is any indication for this. The elderly patient may be confused, and wandering fingers can interfere with the wound or drains. The suction drains are removed when drainage has ceased, usually three or four days after operation.

When the patient returns to the ward the surgeon must have absolute confidence that the operation is secure; that the fracture presents no problem; and the patient may walk forthwith. Therefore it is unnecessary to have more than a simple air permeable adhesive dressing on the wound; the next day the patient gets up and walks, despite the drainage bottles or bags, which can be tied to the walking frame (or put in the dressing gown pocket). This exercise must be part of the routine of the treatment of all patients; there should be no reservations in the mind of any of those looking after them that early walking is wrong or dangerous, because such unspoken anxiety is quickly sensed by the patient. In fact, it is more dangerous not to get the patient out of bed at once, provided the surgery is of the highest quality, because the risk of deep vein thrombosis is reduced and other morbidity, including bedsores, avoided.

During this time the relatives should be seen by the ward sister and the medical social worker to obtain an accurate assessment of the home and circumstances of the patient. The assessment of the patient in the ward continues by day and particularly by night, when any occasional incontinence, confusion, or anxieties become more obvious. If incontinence occurs after operation, despite treatment by hourly bladder discipline, the patient should again undergo catheterisation.

At this stage after the operation the most severely ill patients are transferred to the geriatric orthopaedic unit.

Geriatric orthopaedic unit

The geriatric orthopaedic unit is an ordinary ward with a nursing establishment for acute medicine. That the patients are geriatric increases rather than decreases the workload, not because they are in bed but for the very opposite reason: all patients are up and dressed daily.

In the unit the patient comes under the day to day care of the geriatric physician and his medical staff. The essential feature of the unit is the weekly ward round, which both physician and surgeon and all members of the team attend, including the junior medical staff, the ward sister, physiotherapist, occupational therapist, medical social worker, and the ward secretary. The round eliminates paper work among the members of the team, with its inherent delay. A comprehensive programme is drawn up for all patients, covering either only the next week or the period after the patient's discharge. All patients in the unit dress themselves each day and walk. There is no place in a geriatric orthopaedic unit for the bedridden patient. The unit is geared to the patient partaking in the activities of daily living to the best extent possible; clothes and shoes are therefore kept at the bedside. The occupational therapist instructs and supervises dressing and other activities in close cooperation with the physiotherapist, who treats – and teaches to walk – each patient as necessary. It is most important to realise that an old person dressed feels "up" whereas in a dressing gown she may feel that she should be in bed.

Meanwhile in the acute orthopaedic ward those elderly patients not otherwise ill are discharged without needing to stay in the unit, either home, to a low intensity nursing unit, or to convalescent home.

Medical assessment

The medical assessment of a patient transferred to the geriatric orthopaedic unit has to be comprehensive because the average geriatric patient, especially when frail and senile, usually has several other conditions to be diagnosed and treated. These ailments, including simple anaemia, all impinge on the well being of the patient and her ability to regain independence. The most common medical conditions seen are cardiovascular disease, urinary infections, renal failure, poor sight, and pulmonary and cerebrovascular disease. Psychiatric disorders occur in about 20 % of patients, but these are not necessarily severe and are often sporadic, associated with the sudden admission to hospital with all its fears and strangeness.

Some conditions, such as vertebrobasilar insufficiency, may cause the patient to topple backward when walking, and this tendency may be exacerbated by a walking frame, whereas a frame with wheels eliminates the repeated neck flexion and extension which occurs each time the ordinary walking frame is lifted forward.

When a patient complains of persistent pain, particularly after a hip operation, this invariably indicates that all is not well locally, and full assessment will find a cause. It must never be thought that the patient is complaining unduly. Only when the cause has been found and put right can rehabilitation proceed. Similarly, some patients fail to progress in walking because the operation is not secure and the feeling of instability caused by this is sufficient to deter progress.

At the weekly ward round, and in all daily routines, the patient must be fully involved; often slight deafness or confusion sets patients apart from a discussion on their well being. Patients who do not understand may become frightened, confused, and uncooperative. The enfeebled geriatric patient needs reassurance not only that she will go home but also that she will not go until she is ready. This restores calm and the wish to progress. There are few old people who, given such assurance, do not want to go home.

The psychogeriatrician may be of inestimable help in disturbed or mentally confused patients, particularly those who have a reversed sleep rhythm, being stuporous by day and lively, noisy, and shouting at night. If such patients are treated early the outlook can be very good and in a short time their normal behaviour allows them to continue with the rehabilitation programme with little or no interruption.

Most patients are in the geriatric orthopaedic unit for some three to four weeks; most have then regained their normal level of independence but some may have a medical condition needing further care in a geriatric progressive care ward. A few patients fail to achieve independence and, after careful deliberation, are accepted for long term stay by the consultant geriatrician. This should never happen because surgical complications render the patient incapable of walking. This again emphasises the importance of having a surgical technique that gives the lowest possible complication or failure rate.

Elective procedures

Osteoarthritis in the elderly may destroy independence very quickly because of insecurity and pain. Osteoarthritis of the knee may make patients fall or feel so insecure that they cannot trust themselves with their ordinary activities and, therefore, have to leave their homes and seek some other form of sheltered accommodation. Pain may be so severe that it interferes with rest, and the inactivity that it imposes either causes other intercurrent conditions or prevents the patient looking after herself properly. Therefore, because arthritis is such a pernicious destroyer of independence in the elderly and because it slowly worsens, the patient will become more incapacitated and will have to leave home, so operation is best done early. Many old people still fear a visit to hospital for such an operation and will procrastinate too long, but, because nowadays so many of their friends or relatives have had operations for fractures, it is becoming very much more easy to persuade an old person to have a replacement arthroplasty.

The two arthroplasties that are in great favour at the moment are that of a hip and of a knee. There are many different forms of prosthesis with which to replace these joints, but for the older person a technique should always be chosen that allows the patient to walk immediately. Prolonged bed rest after a replacement procedure can undo all the good in general that the operation has done locally.

The old patient is worried not by the loss of a full range of movement but by the loss of function commensurate with his general activity in his declining years. It is far better for the patient to achieve independence and a speedy return home than to have a prolonged course of treatment to obtain ranges of movement that he does not need in his normal life. Therefore, if the patient can dress, do up shoelaces, walk up stairs, cook, sweep, and get on a bus with no pain or discomfort the operation is highly successful, even if movement in the joint concerned is not full. Striving to regain this loss by physiotherapy is unnecessary.

Venous thrombosis

As at any other age, venous thrombosis will occur in the elderly, but bed rest is undoubtedly a significant inducement of this condition so, again, the sooner the patient is up the less chance is there of a deep vein thrombosis with its possible serious consequence of pulmonary embolism. Should venous thrombosis occur and be considered both progressive and liable to embolise, then anticoagulants can be used, but in the elderly the control may be more difficult than in younger people. If the patient is started on heparin, however, and then continues on warfarin this appears to be tolerated well but must be very carefully controlled.

Some general considerations

The elderly respond well to operations, which should not be long deferred. Whereas in the healthy adult conservative treatment is to be encouraged for such fractures in the femoral or tibial shafts, in the elderly proper and secure internal fixation is always indicated when it can be achieved. An ankle fracture should also be fixed to allow the patient to walk at once, even if in a walking plaster. Even an unstable fracture of the humeral shaft should be internally fixed to allow quick independence.

Fractures of the pelvis and vertebral bodies in old people are almost always stable and should be treated by early walking. To tell the patient that the "backbone has been broken" fills them with alarm; instead a careful explanation that there will be some pain because of "heavy bruising of the bone" and advice that, despite this, the general condition will be better if the patient is up allay fear and give confidence. Mild analgesics should be given freely. Once the patient can sit up in bed – usually in a day or two – it is as comfortable to sit in a chair; the latter is no more painful than standing and the patient is quick to achieve walking.

Lumbar stenosis

The elderly suffer from lumbar stenosis, which is insidious and progressive. The symptoms are bizarre, and physical signs may be completely absent. Patients will complain of weakness of the legs, which causes them to stop walking after a certain distance. They may have difficulty in saying what they would do if there was no chair handy on which to sit and when questioned the patients are not always very clear on what actually happens. They may have peculiar sensory symptoms, such as hot water running up the leg, indescribable aching or pain, and in general a feeling of unreality in the legs – all of which may be revealed in a carefully taken history.

The best investigation for this condition is computed tomography of the lumbar canal, which will show the narrowing almost invariably caused by thickening of the facet articulations impinging on the canal, so that space is reduced. When the patient sits the flexion of the lumbar spine increases the space, so this investigation should be performed after standing or walking. Treatment is by wide decompression, and, again, if this is done with a suitable technique but without actual spinal fusion there is no reason for the patient to stay in bed after the operation.

Pathological fractures and paraplegia

Pathological fractures lend themselves to internal fixation. If metastatic deposits in a femur have so weakened the bone that a fracture is imminent prophylactic intramedullary nailing relieves pain and prevents a catastrophe. Done through the knee the operation takes only a few minutes; the hole made between the femoral condyles through which the nail is passed up the shaft is plugged with cement. Other pathological fractures, whether imminent or present, should be dealt with by a similarly active approach; for thereafter radiotherapy is facilitated because there is no pain and no plaster cast. Because the patient may have only a short while to live it is most important that the quality of what little life remains should be satisfactory.

Paraplegia from metastases is not very common but must be recognised early if treatment is to be of help. The elderly patient who attends with either early paresis or a full blown paraplegia should be treated as acute emergency because if the paresis proceeds to a paraplegia and the paraplegia remains for more than a few hours control of the bladder will be lost and it may not be regained however good the treatment. Therefore any patient in whom paraplegia is present or likely to occur should be given an immediate myelogram after routine radiographs, which will probably show some bone disease. Whether or not the site of the primary tumour is known, the myelogram will show the level of the block if one is present. If no block to the dye in the theca is seen this means that the arterial supply has been damaged and laminectomy and decompression will be of no avail. Once the level of the block is known a full decompression can be done. If this is achieved within a few hours of the onset bladder control will either be maintained or hopefully restored, but if the delay is longer the damage to bladder control is often permanent.

Arteriosclerosis

Once arteriosclerosis is so severe that symptoms are occurring in the legs the prognosis is poor. Therefore if it is possible to preserve the limb for long enough amputation may not be necessary because the normal course of the condition ends the patient's life before avascularity of the limb occurs. To achieve this intermittent venous occlusion by machines which pulsate an inflatable legging and which can be used at home are of great value and may preserve sufficient oxygenation of the leg so that it remains satisfactory.

Nevertheless, amputations do sometimes have to be performed

and, because of the poor prognosis, early walking and consequent early discharge from hospital are essential.

The operation is mentally and surgically traumatic and it may have followed an attempt to preserve the leg by vascular surgery. Understandably the old person dreads the loss of a leg and its consequences, which are an obvious loss of independence. The sooner therefore that the patient can walk again the better. Moreover, if the patient can see the new limb – of whatever type – by the bedside at, or soon after, the time of amputation many anxieties may be allayed. At one or two weeks all geriatric amputees should have the means to walk, whether on a sophisticated artificial leg or a simple early walking aid.

Conclusions

In this short description of geriatric orthopaedics I have emphasised the intensive methods needed to give total care to the aged so that they may continue to enjoy an active and independent life. Geriatric patients are dignified in their acceptance of the inevitable end. They do not ask for longevity. They may at times seem anxious, frail, and disheartened; too often this is because they do not understand what is happening. To them it is not existence that matters but its quality. As in all medicine, the aim of all concerned in their treatment must be the return of function, but, in the elderly, this means a return to independence.

Endocrine disorders in the elderly

PETER J SLEIGHT

The endocrine diseases of the elderly are the same as those found in younger people. Presentation is often atypical, however, and modified by concurrent disease. Biochemical tests may be affected by ill health or multiple drug treatment. Hormonal changes do occur with age but it is not clear whether they are a cause of the aging process itself.

Diabetes mellitus

Most elderly diabetics are non-insulin dependent. They are usually obese. The onset of the disease is often insidious, and symptoms such as tiredness, weight loss, and deterioration in vision are non-specific and easily put down to "getting old." Polyuria, especially at night, and polydypsia may not occur until blood sugar concentrations have reached high values because of declining glomerular filtration rate with age.

A neurological complication may be the first sign of the disease. Usually this is a peripheral sensory neuropathy, but ocular palsies, amyotrophy, autonomic neuropathy (causing postural hypotension), impotence, and bladder dysfunction all occur. Infections, especially of the skin, chest, and urinary tract, are common. Gastrointestinal symptoms include constipation (due to dehydration), diarrhoea (autonomic neuropathy), abdominal pain, and sometimes polyphagia. Visual disturbances may be due to refractive changes (related to hyperglycaemia), cataracts, or maculopathy. Vascular disease is likely in elderly diabetics, and patients may present with myocardial infarction, cerebrovascular disease, or ischaemic legs.

Ketoacidosis may occur for the first time in the very old, and hyperosmolar, hyperglycaemic non-ketotic coma is largely confined to the elderly.

Diagnosis

Glycosuria is the simplest screening test. Confirmatory evidence in patients with characteristic symptoms is provided by a fasting blood sugar value greater than 8 mmol/l (145 mg/100ml) or a random (or two hour postprandial) value greater than 11 mmol/l (200 mg/100 ml). Raised blood sugar concentrations below these limits indicate impaired glucose tolerance. This occurs naturally with aging,[1] but there is an increased chance of developing overt diabetes and a much increased risk of coronary heart disease in this group.[2] Blood glucose concentrations should be measured in all confused or comatose elderly patients.

Management

The aims of treatment in the elderly diabetic are to prevent the problems of severe hyperglycaemia and hypoglycaemia and to minimise complications of the disease. The desire for meticulous control must be balanced against the patient's quality of life. For most elderly people with mild diabetes testing urine before breakfast is a sufficient check on control. The percentage of glycosylated haemoglobin gives a measure of overall control, but this also increases with age.[3]

Diet should be related as far as possible to the patient's present eating habits. Adequate education is essential and needs to be reinforced. Responsible relatives or friends or the practice nurse may need to be involved. In obese patients the aim should be a reduction in energy intake. Carbohydrate food should be unrefined and high in fibre. Total fat content should be reduced with the inclusion of more unsaturated fat. An adequate intake of protein, minerals, and vitamins is important, but patients may resist the suggestion because of the expense. Food should be taken regularly, especially by patients taking oral hypoglycaemic agents or insulin. Patients who respond to dietary restriction must be kept under regular supervision, since relapse can occur because of either dietary indiscretion or worsening of diabetes.

Exercise is very important and should be encouraged whatever the age of the patient.

Oral hypoglycaemic agents are indicated if, after a few weeks, it is obvious that dietary control is not working. Long acting tablets, such as chlorpropamide or glibenclamide, carry the risk of nocturnal hypoglycaemia if the dose is too high or the evening meal omitted. Shorter acting drugs – for example, tolbutamide – are preferable but need to be taken two or three times a day, and may cause problems with compliance. Drug interactions are a problem, and

183

hypoglycaemia may be potentiated by commonly used drugs such as co-trimoxazole, β blockers, aspirin, and other non-steroidal anti-inflammatory drugs. In overweight diabetics unresponsive to diet the biguanide metformin may be considered.

Insulin is necessary to treat ketoacidotic and hyperosmolar coma. It may also be needed temporarily at times of stress (infections, surgery). It should also be used permanently if diet and tablets have failed to give adequate control. A single daily injection is preferable – either of an intermediate acting insulin alone or of an intermediate acting insulin combined with a shorter acting one. Errors in the use of insulin are common.[4] Impaired vision, forgetfulness, or lack of manual dexterity often make it necessary for another person to give the injection.

Hypoglycaemia – Patient education and cautious drug treatment should help to prevent hypoglycaemia. Warning symptoms may not be noticed because of neuroglycopenia or concurrent β blocker administration. Hypoglycaemia should be considered in any elderly diabetic who presents with failing mental function, confusion, convulsions, hypothermia, or transient hemiparesis. Treatment of hypoglycaemic coma is by intravenous glucose or, often more conveniently, 1 mg of intramuscular glucagon.

Visual failure – Maculopathy with exudates and oedema may compromise central vision. Laser therapy is the treatment of choice. Cataract extraction should always be considered whatever the age of the patient, and early ophthalmic referral enables the state of the fundus to be documented before the cataract matures.

Foot care – Poor eyesight and mental impairment lead to an increased risk of injury to feet already suffering from peripheral vascular insufficiency and neuropathy. Loss of the ability to walk leads to loss of independence. Sensible footwear, frequent washing, the use of skin softeners, and avoidance of hot water bottles should all be emphasised. Regular visits to the chiropodist are essential.

Thyroid disease

Thyroid disease becomes commoner with age, but atypical presentation and problems in interpreting thyroid function test results may cause diagnostic difficulties.

Thyrotoxicosis

Only a small proportion of patients have classical symptoms, and female preponderance is less pronounced than in younger patients.[5] Toxic multinodular goitre or solitary autonomous nodules are found more often than Graves' disease, and a high proportion of patients have no palpable thyroid enlargement at all.[6]

Weight loss, proximal myopathy, or cardiovascular abnormalities such as atrial fibrillation or cardiac failure may predominate and be associated with an apathetic rather than a hyperkinetic state.[7] There is often a relative absence of tachycardia.

In obvious thyrotoxicosis a high serum thyroxine concentration is diagnostic. In the elderly concurrent disease or drug treatment may cause changes in thyroid binding proteins, and the free thyroxine index is a more accurate test than measuring protein bound thyroxine. Serum triiodothyronine values should be measured in patients with clinical features suggestive of thyrotoxicosis but with no increase in serum thyroxine concentrations. If the diagnosis is still in doubt autonomy of the thyroid gland may be shown by failure of thyroid stimulating hormone concentrations to rise after intravenous injection of thyroid releasing hormone. It has been suggested that hyperthyroidism should not be dismissed as a cause of otherwise unexplained atrial fibrillation without a thyroid releasing hormone test being performed.[8] Assays of free thyroid hormone and thyroxine binding globulin are becoming more widely available. They are more specific but still subject to drug interaction.

Radioactive iodine is the treatment of choice in elderly patients unless pressure symptoms from a large goitre dictate surgery. Antithyroid drugs (such as neomercazole) or β blockers may control symptoms until radiation is effective. Some physicians deliberately give a large initial dose of iodine-131 to induce hypothyroidism and then continue with thyroid replacement therapy.

Hypothyroidism

Hypothyroidism is often difficult to recognise in the elderly. Biochemical screening of patients admitted to geriatric units has found an incidence of 2–3%.[9] The incidence in the healthy elderly is, however, much lower than this, and the advantages of wide-scale screening in the elderly are debatable.[10]

Presenting features may point to a psychiatric disorder (depression, confusion), an ear, nose, and throat problem (hoarseness, deafness), or gastrointestinal disease (constipation). Neurological (ataxia, polyneuritis), dermatological (dry skin, facial oedema, hair loss), or haematological (anaemia) manifestations may predominate. It is because presentation is so varied that the disease is overlooked. General slowing up and changes in appearance may be so insidious as to be unnoticed by patients, relatives, and doctor alike.

185

Occasionally a patient presents in myxoedema coma. This tends to be precipitated by cold, drugs, or infection. Most patients are hypothermic, although the number of hypothermic patients who are hypothyroid is relatively small.

Diagnosis of hypothyroidism is made on the basis of a low serum thyroxine value of free thyroxine index associated with a raised thyroid stimulating hormone. Measurement of serum thyroxine concentration alone is not diagnostic because non-thyroidal illness and drug interference can both lower it.

Treatment is with thyroxine. In elderly patients, especially those with cardiovascular disease, an initial dose of 25 μg is satisfactory, increasing to 50 μg after two weeks. The final dose can be titrated using thyroxine and thyroid stimulating hormone measurements. Doses greater than 150 μg daily are unusual and suggest non-compliance.

Hypercalcaemia

Symptomatic hypercalcaemia in the elderly is usually caused by malignant disease. Routine calcium estimations have led to considerable increase in the number of cases of hyperparathyroidism diagnosed, especially in elderly women.[11] Patients aged over 70 with symptoms do improve after parathyroidectomy,[12] but a conservative policy is advisable in the asymptomatic patient.[13]

Hyponatraemia

Inappropriately increased secretion of antidiuretic hormone may occur in a number of conditions, including bronchial carcinoma, chest infections, and hypothyroidism. Diagnosis is suggested by hyponatraemia and a urine osmolality greater than plasma osmolality in a patient who is not hypovolaemic. Symptoms include weakness, confusion, and fitting. Treatment is by fluid restriction or, if this is poorly tolerated, demeclocycline. Far more commonly, the cause of hyponatraemia in the elderly is iatrogenic (diuretic or intravenous fluid therapy).[14]

Oestrogen disorders

Oestrogen deficiency is a factor in the development of osteoporosis and vascular disease in older women. Vaginal atrophy, urinary frequency, and urge incontinence in postmenopausal women may be helped by oral or topical oestrogens. Tamoxifen, an antioestrogen, is now considered to be an appropriate primary treatment for breast cancer in the elderly.[15]

Other endocrine disorders

Features of Cushing's syndrome in the elderly are most commonly caused by steroid therapy. Ectopic adrenocorticotrophic hormone production (usually from bronchial carcinoma) produces a clinical picture characterised by hypokalaemia, weakness, and hypertension. The classical features of Cushing's syndrome may not have time to develop.

Hyperaldosteronism usually occurs as a secondary phenomenon in patients with congestive cardiac failure, hepatic, and renal disease.

The low reported incidence of non-thyroidal or non-diabetic endocrine disease in the very old is probably due to lack of clinical suspicion, a desire not to overinvestigate, and the relative rarity of the condition anyway.

1 Davidson MB. The effect of ageing on carbohydrate metabolism; a review of the English literature and a practical approach to the diagnosis of diabetes mellitus in the elderly. *Metabolism* 1979; **28**: 688–705.

2 Keen H, Fuller JH. The epidemiology of diabetes. In: Exton-Smith N, Caird FI, eds. *Metabolic and nutritional disorders in the elderly.* Bristol: J Wright, 1980: 146–60.

3 Graf RJ, Halter JB, Porte D. Glycosylated hemoglobin in normal subjects and subjects with maturity onset diabetes. Evidence for a saturable system in men. *Diabetes* 1978; **27**: 834–9.

4 Watkins JD, Roberts ED, Williams TF, Martin DA, Coyle VC. Observation of medication errors made by diabetic patients in the home. *Diabetes* 1967; **16**: 882–5.

5 Kawabe T, Komya I, Endo T, Koizumi Y, Yanvada T. Hyperthyroidism in the elderly *J Am Geriatr Soc* 1979; **27**: 152–5.

6 Davis PJ, Davis B. Hyperthyroidism in patients over the age of 60 years *Medicine* (Baltimore) 1974; **53**: 161–81.

7 Thomas FB, Mazzaferri EL, Skillman TG. Apathetic thyrotoxicosis: a distinctive clinical and laboratory entity. *Ann Intern Med* 1970; **72**: 679–85.

8 Forfar JC, Miller HC, Toft AD. Occult thyrotoxicosis: a correctable course of "idiopathic" atrial fibrillation. *Am J Cardiol* 1979; **44**: 9–12.

9 Bahemuka M, Hodkinson HM. Screening for hypothyroidism in elderly inpatients. *Br Med J* 1975; ii: 601–3.

10 Heikoff LE, Luxenberg J, Fergenbaum LZ. Low yield of screening for hypothyroidism in healthy elderly. *J Am Geriatr Soc* 1984; **32**: 616–7.

11 Munday GR, Cove DH, Frisken R. Primary hyperparathyroidism: changes in the pattern of clinical presentation. *Lancet* 1980; i: 1317–20.

12 Heath DA, Wright AD, Barnes AD, Oates GD, Dorricott NJ. Surgical treatment of primary hyperthyroidism in the elderly. *Br Med J* 1980; **280**: 1406–8.

13 Pearson MW. Asymptomatic primary hyperparathyroidism in the elderly – a review. *Age Ageing* 1984; **13**: 1–5.

[14] Sunderam SG, Mankikar GD. Hyponatraemia in the elderly. *Age Ageing* 1983; **12**: 77–80.
[15] Allan SG, Rodger A, Smyth JF, Leonard RCF, Chetty U, Forrest APM. Tamoxifen as primary treatment of breast cancer in elderly or frail patients: a practical management. *Br Med J* 1985; **290**: 358.

Index